THE MEDICAL
JUNGLE

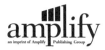

www.amplifypublishing.com

The Medical Jungle: A Pioneering Surgeon's Battle to Revolutionize Vascular Care and Challenge the Medical Mafia

For more information, please contact:
Amplify Publishing, an imprint of Amplify Publishing Group
620 Herndon Parkway, Suite 320
Herndon, VA 20170
info@amplifypublishing.com

Library of Congress Control Number: 2022904248

CPSIA Code: PRV0822A

ISBN-13:978-1-63755-262-9

Printed in the United States

For Carol—your loving support, intelligence, wisdom, care, and encouragement are unparalleled. Life would never be the same without you.

THE MEDICAL
JUNGLE

**A Pioneering Surgeon's Battle
to Revolutionize Vascular Care
and Challenge the Medical Mafia**

FRANK J. VEITH, MD

with Glenn Plaskin

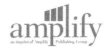

amplify
an imprint of Amplify Publishing Group

CONTENTS

Preface: Against the Grain 1

CHAPTER 1 ACCIDENTAL DESTINY 11

CHAPTER 2 SEASONED IN THE ARMY, LAUNCHED INTO THE LAB 23

CHAPTER 3 BREATH IN, BREATH OUT: INNOVATIONS IN
LUNG TRANSPLANTATION 35

CHAPTER 4 THE ART OF LIMB SALVAGE 55

CHAPTER 5 THE ENDOVASCULAR REVOLUTION 81

CHAPTER 6 VALIANT CRUSADE: RECOGNIZING VASCULAR SURGERY AS
AN INDEPENDENT SPECIALTY 119

CHAPTER 7 ALL UNDER ONE TENT: THE VEITHSYMPOSIUM 145

CHAPTER 8 MENTORSHIP: THE LASTING LEGACY 167

Epilogue: Looking Forward 205

Acknowledgments 209

Appendix 213

AGAINST THE GRAIN

In the life and death business of vascular surgery, there is no room to make any mistakes, so I always took my work seriously—to say the least. In fact, by the time I became Chief of Vascular Surgery at New York's Montefiore Medical Center and Albert Einstein College of Medicine, my exacting standards had earned me a dubious nickname.

To some residents and junior staff, I was ominously known as the White Shark—an intimidating presence who was constructively critical to a fault. As one of my most prominent trainees remarked: "In those days, he lived up to his nickname. He would bite your head off before you could yell 'get out of the water.'"

But I never really saw myself that way. True, in my role as teacher and mentor, I had to be strict in and out of the operating room, more attuned to a patient's needs than a young doctor's feelings. I would painstakingly watch (and correct) every throw of an anastomotic stitch until it was perfect. The demands of my role required total confidence and an assertive personality.

Yet years earlier, as a medical student at Cornell and later as a resident at Harvard and the Peter Bent Brigham Hospital (the Brigham), I was anything but a shark. I was more of a minnow—extremely shy. I was someone who listened carefully, worried a lot, and was somewhat intimidated by my superiors.

I rarely asked questions. I never volunteered. Instead, I would sit in the back of the auditorium and hope that I never got called on. Many of us felt like enlisted men in the service—total subordinates to the senior surgeons, never dreaming that some among us would one day step into their shoes.

But as my enchantment with vascular surgery surged, my devotion to the field evolved into a lifelong obsession. By the time I was in the army, given the opportunity to do numerous operations on my own, my shyness quickly subsided. And by the time I was chief resident at the Brigham, my confidence matched my responsibility. Somehow, I had grown into being someone I never expected.

As Maya Angelou once said, "If you are always trying to be normal, you will never know how amazing you can be." I truly believe that. In medicine, there are physicians who lead conventional lives, going with the flow, following the traditional path of seeing patients, making appearances at medical conferences, writing a paper or two, and playing golf or tennis on weekends.

But there are others who become iconoclasts, who go against the grain and challenge current wisdom. They put their necks on the line to defy the predictable and strike out in innovative ways. As pioneers, they tackle challenges that others have either fumbled or thought were impossible.

That's what this book is all about: GOING AGAINST THE GRAIN, often overcoming resistance or fighting back against opposition from some of the dangerous beasts that populate the medical jungle. To do this, you must think outside the box rather than following the herd. You must not bend to other people's notions of how things should be done. You don't simply follow existing protocols or guidelines. You're a leader. You're a nonconformist. You have to survive and function in an often hostile, jungle-like environment.

That was me, trying to get people to realize that the impossible was possible. And as you'll read, I have paid for that in some distressing ways. There were many days when I was greeted with skepticism, disdain, and professional jealousy. At times, I was even ridiculed and deemed a "crazy man." Yet most of the things I advocated later became the standard of care (particularly true with lung transplantation, transformational limb salvage, and endovascular procedures).

For decades, it was a struggle to get funding, support, or peer approval for our innovations. This was true particularly at Montefiore Medical Center in the Bronx, which was dwarfed by more prestigious institutions like the Mayo Clinic, Massachusetts General Hospital, Columbia-Presbyterian Medical Center, the Brigham, or Johns Hopkins.

Yet through it all, we somehow managed to turn Montefiore into a Mecca for vascular surgery that superseded other institutions. How? By leading an aggressive approach to limb salvage and becoming the first vascular physician group in the US to perform less invasive endovascular aortic aneurysm repair. This breakthrough, a total team effort, made it possible to treat or replace any medium-sized or large artery in the body in a brand-new way. And when we did it, there were many who attacked us out of disbelief or jealousy. As you'll see, there were witch hunts and hidden agendas—storylines that were positively Shakespearian. I would hear back-channel chatter from competing hospitals: "This guy is nuts. He's a maverick working at a third-rate institution in the Bronx. How is he going to accomplish that!?"

As you will read, the experience of all this backbiting taught me some crucial lessons about the less attractive aspects of human nature. I saw resentment born of competition lead to cruelty and poor decisions. I was, at times, astonished and admittedly hurt by the furtive efforts of others to thwart our worthy pursuits, just because competing factions wanted to get the credit or get ahead. I learned that the best way to deal with all the ugly qualities of professional jealousy is to shut them out and continue your mission, no matter what.

So, over six decades as a vascular surgeon, I kept pushing forward in my research and experimentation, authoring more than a thousand original articles and chapters in medical journals and books that maintained forward momentum. True, I could have gone into private practice, following the path of other surgeons who were making millions of dollars. Instead, I was committed to an academic career, accepting less money to do what I thought was right for me. I wanted to make a difference, and that's where this story begins.

In the pages ahead, there are six primary areas that form the pillars of our story, landmarks in my medical career that I consider unusual. These are experiences that I hope may inspire others to explore new ground, no matter what their profession.

First, you will read about my fifteen-year mission to overcome the major obstacles that prevented lung transplantation from being a practical therapeutic treatment.

We had to confute the notion that the lung was the poor sister of transplantation, that the procedure was fated to fail. Traditionally, a lung taken out of a donor was thought to have a high level of vascular resistance in the recipient (for reasons to be discussed). But in our protocols, we created a surgical technique that allowed normal blood flow at a low level of vascular resistance in the recipient, making single-lung transplantation in a variety of conditions totally feasible. You'll see how our work was ultimately blocked by the impossibility of getting donor lungs in New York City because vying institutions refused to share them. Ultimately though, we made human lung transplantation a reality, performing seven single-lung transplants in desperately ill patients.

Second, you will see how I devoted a huge amount of my time to saving lower limbs that were afflicted with gangrene, cases that would require a major amputation in other institutions. The wisdom of the day in the late sixties and seventies was that any surgical attempt to improve the blood supply to a gangrenous foot caused more harm than good. As such, lower limbs with toe or foot gangrene due to poor blood supply were routinely treated by below-knee amputation. But we challenged that widely held assumption and developed all sorts of techniques for treating those threatened limbs, eventually saving over 90 percent of them.

Yet when we presented our results to prestigious learned societies, they believed that "those guys in the Bronx" were unhinged, or that we were not presenting the data accurately. Today, almost all of our techniques have been proven successful and are in general use worldwide.

Third, as mentioned, we were the first to repair aneurysms as well as obstructed arteries with less invasive endovascular procedures that did not require open operations. Everybody thought we were out of our minds on that one too. But our breakthrough came in 1992, when (in partnership with Juan Parodi, an Argentinian vascular surgeon) we performed the first endovascular repair of an aneurysm of the aorta in the US. It was accomplished with a surgeon-made endovascular graft placed within the blood vessel. The same technique also allowed us to effectively treat most ruptured aortic aneurysms, as well as other arterial obstructions and injuries, such as stab or gunshot wounds.

I am proud to say that our initial procedures created an endovascular revolution that spread throughout the world. Today, 85 percent to 90 percent of all blood vessel pathology is treated endovascularly, a technique we originally promoted against intense opposition.

Fourth, and most controversially, you will read about how I led the fight to make vascular surgery a distinct and independent specialty. Traditionally, the field of vascular surgery was a subordinate or subservient subspecialty within a department of general or cardiac surgery. In this arrangement, vascular surgery was the poor sister, having to appeal to our "fathers" in the parent department to get needed resources like staff, space, money, and equipment.

As endovascular techniques evolved, my belief was that we deserved our own separate specialty niche. Why? Because general surgeons simply didn't perform procedures on blood vessels as well as committed vascular surgery specialists did. Inevitably, we produced far better results and lower mortality rates, which justified our being an independent specialty.

In the late nineties and early 2000s, a few colleagues and I pushed hard for independence within the structure of US medicine. We also lobbied Congress and generated significant media attention, with published articles in the *Wall Street Journal* and elsewhere. Our activism was divisive within vascular surgery and opposed by many. The position that we advocated was deemed revolutionary and *against the grain* of established organized medical specialization.

Despite a passionate effort to assert our independence, we sadly lost the fight. This was due to strong opposition from general surgery and its American Board of Surgery (ABS) and the American Board of Medical Specialties (ABMS), an unfair, self-serving, cartel-like structure in US-organized medicine. We were also opposed by some individuals in our own specialty—those who valued career advancement over what was best for patients and vascular surgery as a vocation.

Bottom line: after a thirty-year career at Montefiore that was successful in every way—academically, clinically, and financially (in terms of patients attracted, research achievements, and grants procured)—I was terminated because of my efforts to challenge and change the structure of organized medicine (which I have come to think of as the medical equivalent of the Sicilian Mafia) to establish a new independent specialty.

To this day the fight goes on. And, regrettably, the same dominance of self-interests over patient and specialty interests still appears to be operative.

Fifth, I will tell you about how and why I led the development of the so-called VEITHsymposium—an international continuing medical education event that provides vascular surgeons and all vascular specialists with updates on the latest advances, changing concepts in diagnosis, pressing controversies, and new techniques.

It all began in the early 1970s when I helped Dr. Henry Haimovici start a small meeting in New York that attracted less than a hundred attendees. After a few years, I took over and expanded this program. I was fortunate: as vascular surgery grew and matured as a specialty, the event exploded in size and importance. Today, the VEITHsymposium is arguably the largest vascular meeting in the world, attracting approximately five thousand attendees annually.

Sixth, but not least, you will read about what I consider my biggest career achievement, my commitment to mentorship and career promotion of others. For anyone in a leadership position, giving back is a huge gift and responsibility.

Through all the advancements described here, it was never, ever a one-man show. My colleagues at Montefiore were a band of brothers and sisters, like a marine company who always stood up for one another, even when we were demeaned by jealous superiors or ill-motivated administrators. We shared everything, both the blame and the credit. When you're a leader, you have to make other people great. It has to be *we*, not *me*.

It was a tradition that the renowned heart surgeon Michael DeBakey always practiced as he mentored his surgical trainees from around the world. Promoting colleagues in the end always promotes you. I became driven to make my associates successful, not only by training them, but by advancing their careers with the sharing of lead authorship on articles and financial rewards, the distribution of interesting patients, partnering on research, and more.

Perhaps I did it for selfish reasons, to create a legacy that would live on as long as my trainees carried *their* work forward, then passing it on to progeny of their own. I often hope that, even after everything else I have been able to do is forgotten, the legacy of my trainees and associates will endure and remain relevant. I feel paternally toward them, and I am delighted that so many have become leaders in the world of vascular surgery.

There you have it: the six fundamentals that compose *The Medical Jungle*, a book about the stories, principles, and philosophies that helped me build my own success and hopefully help in shaping the future success of others.

My mission in this book is to guide anyone in or out of medicine to achieve prominence and excellence, by proving that they too can thrive in a high-performance field that may sometimes feel like a swimming pool full of sharks. My hope is that any physician or professional will have the courage to go against the grain themselves in whatever way serves their cause best. Perhaps someone else will be inspired by my example to push forward, even in an unpopular crusade.

I always tell young people to choose a topic within their specialty that *isn't* attractive, something off the beaten path that hasn't been done before or that folks think can't be done. It might seem as if you're going in the wrong direction. And you might experience pushback as I did. But you have to persevere. I think of Winston Churchill when he proclaimed, "Never, never, never, never, never give up!" That's been pretty much my motto, not accepting defeat, even when defeat loomed before me.

In the end, the lessons ahead speak to the traits of success—a high energy level, persistence, hard work, building a team, and of course, just plain luck.

FRANK J. VEITH, MARCH 2022

CHAPTER ONE

ACCIDENTAL DESTINY

P erhaps medicine was always in my genes.

My mother, Elsie, was a nurse who served during WWI. Tragically, she died in childbirth, leaving my shocked father alone. Dad immediately hired a registered nurse named Joan O'Sullivan, a strong, funny, positive person. From the moment we came home from the hospital, she cared for me as if she were my own mother. Ultimately, she stayed on with our family and married my father when I was five.

Mom was a staunch Irish Catholic, born in Ireland and trained in London. She worked as a field nurse in the Black and Tan War, fighting for Ireland against England before coming to the US. By the time I was born in August 1931, she was working at Doctor's Hospital in New York City.

As I think back on it now, her nursing work might have nudged me in the direction of a medical career. But it was my favorite paternal uncle, James, a dentist, who was always talking to me about the attraction of being a physician. Uncle James was also an avid outdoorsman who passed on to me his love of sports.

During our outings together fishing and hunting in Maine and upstate New York, he'd tell me about his best friend, Dr. Thompson, a general surgeon whom he greatly admired. Both of them were always touting the benefits of being a doctor. To an impressionable kid like me, it sounded kind of magical.

Of course, as I developed, I really didn't know what my future would be. But these influences definitely mattered, in addition to the odd coincidence of having two mothers who were nurses and an uncle who nudged me in the direction of medicine. All I know is that medicine seemed like a challenging and worthwhile thing to do.

I certainly never gravitated toward the profession of my father, Frank Veith Sr., who was a New York City lawyer specializing in estate planning, tax, and real estate. I later went into medicine in part because I was turned off by my father always coming home with so much paperwork to do. I never wanted that burden. (Ironically, in later years I did much more writing and academic paperwork than he ever did—penning thousands of articles, chapters, abstracts, and grant proposals as my career unfolded.)

Dad, who was a second-generation German, was a quiet, capable, more introverted person, less outgoing than either my mother or his brother James. It was my mother who was the dominating force, the disciplinarian at home, not my easygoing dad.

In fact, my father was amazingly nonaggressive for an attorney. He was never pushy, but he conveyed a clear example of right and wrong and a vital sense of ethics, a quality that would become an intrinsic part of my personality later on when I went against the grain of the Medical Mafia to fight for what I thought was right.

But all that controversy was eons away for a kid growing up in on the Upper East Side of Manhattan near the Guggenheim Museum and Central Park at Eighty-Eighth Street. It was an upper-middle-class upbringing, though we were conservative and never showy. My parents were in a contented marriage and gave me a rather carefree, uneventful childhood.

As an only child, I guess I got used to the limelight, which may have been another psychological factor that led to my managerial sense, the feeling that I liked being in charge of things, which every surgeon requires. With me being the center of their world, my parents spoiled me a bit, yes, and treated me like an adult. I had the good fortune of always being included in their weekend and seasonal getaways, summer vacations to Maine and winter trips to Florida. I enjoyed swimming, canoeing, fishing, and hiking, particularly in Maine. There were family cruises too. This exposure to New York, Florida, and Maine was an advantage not to be taken for granted, a definite asset in expanding my view of the world.

As a kid, I always preferred being outdoors to being stuck inside at school. In fact, during my early years at Public School 6, I was never highly motivated as a student—but I did skip two grades in grammar school, so I must have been okay. Still, my marks were only slightly above average.

By the time my parents enrolled me at Horace Mann, a prestigious high school in Riverdale, I was not particularly outstanding as a student. I was much more interested in playing intramural sports with friends than in book work. Personality-wise, I was always socially shy, though physically outgoing and filled with energy. Despite my desire to get outside and play, I was also interested in current events—especially the battles of the Second World War, which I followed daily in the *New York Times*.

Overall, I remained less than highly motivated from an academic standpoint, yet my dad, a Cornell graduate, wanted me to follow in his footsteps. That didn't seem very likely. Actually, I was told by my high school guidance counselors that I didn't have a chance of getting into an Ivy League college like Cornell due to my average grades and lack of extracurricular activities. I don't remember being active in any club or charity. I didn't have any notable talent, nor did I earn a varsity letter.

Yet I did manage to get into Dad's alma mater. How so? I probably did better on the SAT than I realized. I never knew.

Once I got onto the Ithaca campus, surrounded by all those brainiacs who had earned straight A's in high school, it wasn't long before I had a drastic coming of age. My attitude toward studying was transformed. For the first time in my life, I felt intimidated, fearful that I wasn't going to do very well. I could no longer just get by.

With a vague notion of becoming a doctor, I majored in zoology and pursued a pre-medical curriculum. I buckled down and immersed myself in the animal sciences department. It offered an opportunity to study animal biology and other life sciences, chemistry, animal evolution and development, anatomy, and physiology.

The curriculum at Cornell was extremely flexible, which somewhat whetted my appetite for the *human* kind of medicine too. (I enjoyed performing first aid remedies on family members and fellow students, little things such as removing a splinter from a hand, which gave me a feel for medicine and helping others.)

Still, at this point I wasn't greatly turned on by the idea of becoming a doctor. Why not? I had worked as an orderly at a local hospital during college and found it rather boring. But to a rather immature kid in his late teens with a fascination for animal physiology and anatomy (and no interest in a chemistry major) it seemed like the best option, a career choice by default.

So, after three years of undergraduate work, you might say I sort of stumbled into medical school with mixed feelings. I had worked hard and managed to get top grades, not only in zoology but in all my undergraduate courses. I applied to various medical schools and was accepted at Harvard and Cornell. Unwisely, I chose Cornell because I had won a New York State scholarship and could get a blended AB and MD degree, which was not possible at Harvard Medical School. I would later view this youthful decision as an error because I considered Harvard a better medical school.

In med school I still felt insecure, worried that I might not be able to keep up my grades. But as things turned out, I didn't find the course work that tough. It was hard work for sure, with much memorization, but I was able to master it pretty well.

Still, as I mentioned in the Preface, I was extremely shy in medical school. Because of the formal setting of the classes and the imperious temperament of the professors, I wanted to be as inconspicuous as possible. Trust me, I never went against the grain *then*.

Outside of school, I enjoyed blowing off steam back in the dorm, horsing around with my mates. I especially liked playing touch football in the yard of our dormitory on the East River, establishing a true camaraderie with classmates who had been on college varsity teams. Within the dorm, there was a lot of wrestling. In one of these matches, I remember accidentally pushing the head of one of my classmates right through the flimsy plasterboard walls of the dorm. That sticks in my mind (and in his!), but it was all in good fun and no one got hurt.

After my sophomore year as an undergraduate, I had impulsively decided to volunteer at Cornell for senior ROTC out of a genuine interest in the military and a sense of patriotism. Unlike many kids my age (who were entirely self-focused) this was an avenue that really drew me in. Little did I know that the Korean War would break out while I was undergoing basic infantry summer training. Without question, as new officer trainees, we were ripe candidates to be airlifted to Korea as second lieutenants to reinforce our troops—who were being pushed into the sea at Pusan by the Red Chinese Army.

Fortunately, the order to go was rescinded and I was allowed to return to college and then to med school. Not going to Korea probably saved my life, as the average lifespan of an infantry second lieutenant in battle was about ten minutes! But this attraction to the military definitely foreshadowed what would become my service in the army years later. More on that in a bit.

When I graduated from medical school in 1955, I ranked first in my class—which was a surprise to me, as we were not informed of our grades, although I had been elected to Alpha Omega Alpha, a medical school honorary society. It was now time to choose what to do next. I thought about going into internal medicine—which was considered the more intellectually demanding field back then. However, because I really liked and excelled in the hands-on aspects of animal surgery, I took a surgical internship. (My uncle had told me that general surgeons were the true stars of medicine. That might have been true in 1935, but it certainly is not true today.)

I remember one particular event that nudged me toward surgery. It was the gratifying experience of caring for a patient with a perforated ulcer, seeing him totally cured by a simple operation at which I assisted. Witnessing this positive outcome fueled my resolve to continue on a surgical path.

For my surgical internship, I applied to Massachusetts General, Peter Bent Brigham, and Columbia-Presbyterian Medical Center. Because I wanted to stay close to my parents in New York, I ultimately chose a general surgery internship at Columbia-Presbyterian. But honestly, attending Columbia was another mistake, just as choosing Cornell over Harvard had been. Why? Because the Brigham (again, at Harvard) was a better training program.

At Columbia, the atmosphere was highly competitive, as we were all vying for the top spots and the favor of the attending surgeons. Each of us wanted to be assigned to interesting cases and to participate in surgeries—supervised, of course, by senior residents or an attending physician.

My first experiences as the operating surgeon were procedures like an appendectomy or a hernia repair. Although it was great training, I only stayed at Columbia for one year. When I completed my internship, I received a Berry Plan deferment—meaning I could defer my obligatory military service until I completed my residency training—but this was not possible at Columbia. They required that I go into the army immediately after my internship.

So I obtained a surgical residency position at the Brigham, a teaching affiliate of Harvard Medical School. This institution was renowned for its groundbreaking biomedical research and excellence in treating multiple categories of disease. The Brigham would allow me to use my deferment so that I could complete my training and go into the services as a trained surgeon, not just a general medical officer.

This new beginning in Boston was a defining period in my training and professional life. I spent a total of five years there as a resident surgeon, with two additional years as chief of surgery at a large army hospital in Fort Carson near Colorado Springs.

The history of my surgical training went like this: one year of internship in New York; four years of general surgery residency at the Brigham; two years in the army; capped by a fifth year as chief resident at the Brigham. I then stayed on at the Brigham as the prestigious Arthur Tracy Cabot Research Fellow—working under the future Nobel laureate Dr. Joseph Murray in transplant research. (Dr. Murray and his Brigham colleagues were early world leaders in the exciting field of human kidney transplantation.)

From the start, the Brigham was a fascinating place to be. While it has grown into a 793-bed hospital which draws patients from 120 countries, back in the fifties it was much smaller, with ample chances for a young resident to shine. I felt fortunate to be a junior member of the surgical house staff, as my fellows were all superstars, the top people in their classes from whichever medical school they came from.

Like all surgical internships of the day, it was a pyramidal system, highly competitive. Ten to twelve surgical trainees started as interns or junior residents, and only one finished at the top of the pyramid, all the others having been eliminated or drawn into other specialties. (Today, everyone who starts as an intern can finish their training.) Ultimately, whoever became chief resident in surgery was a lucky guy. It was a very prestigious and important position, because that person became the second most powerful surgeon in the hospital, second only to the chairman or chief of surgery.

The chief resident's duties included running the entire non-private surgical service, training junior residents, picking patients for rounds, inviting guest speakers, organizing important conferences, and much more.

For your time in the sun, you were treated like a king! And then, at the end of a year, it was over. Regrettably, you lost your power and returned to the normal reality of a young surgeon. You were nothing. You were out. And somebody else would come on and become chief resident.

Everyone knew who the real boss was anyway: the chairman of surgery, Dr. Francis Moore, a giant of twentieth-century surgery who had even appeared on the cover of *Time*. Moore was the most prominent surgeon of his day, and had made profound contributions to the understanding of how bodily fluids and electrolytes change during surgery. He was also a trailblazer in the development of organ transplantation and the care of critically ill surgical patients.

He was a perfect role model, someone who did virtually everything well. He was a trailblazing researcher, a charismatic speaker, a wise educator, a brilliant technical surgeon—tops in everything. (He was also a world-class sailor and a skilled accordion player!)

To say the least, Dr. Moore was intimidating. And he liked being in total charge. In fact, I believe that the structure of his surgical department was purposefully designed to maintain his authority and unquestioned leadership. That aside, he was the jewel of the hospital and we were lucky to have him. In my eyes, he was just an all-round great person. Stimulated by his spectacular example, I aspired to be even half the surgeon he was. We all looked up to the mighty Dr. Moore.

As green-behind-the-ears junior surgical residents, our day-to-day relationships were, however, more focused on working with the senior residents and attending staffs. They became mentors to us, unlike the colder approach at Columbia, where staff and residents comprised two different strata, never equals in status or social contact.

As surgical residents at the Brigham, we worked unbelievably hard by today's standards and performed many tasks that would be done today by nurses or technicians. Sometimes it was just the simple lab work, or transporting patients back and forth to the operating room; other times we served as intensivists, staffing both the recovery room and the intensive care unit, providing all services imaginable.

For example, while taking care of sick postoperative cardiac or thoracic surgery patients, you'd be up all night. Why? Back in the late 1950s, ventilators were unreliable so we would end up having to "bag" the patient, i.e., ventilate their lungs manually with a compressible bag, taking turns throughout the entire night, one breath at a time. It was a physically and emotionally exhausting process with a patient's life literally in your hands. No room for error. Even on so-called nights "off," you might only get four hours of sleep, all of it spent in a cramped room or in the hospital corridor.

Though it was a very challenging regimen, it produced endurance and an ability to weather the stressful demands of a surgical career or an ICU, no matter what they might be.

On some nights, we were tasked with hunting down the so-called White Elephant. I'll explain. Before surgeries, patients had to be weighed. At the Brigham, we had a massive portable scale we nicknamed the White Elephant. It was huge and heavy and required two of us to move from one ward to another, usually at 5:30 in the morning before the first operation started.

First, we would have to find the scale, which involved a page operator sending an all-hospital call out. We would eventually deliver it, weigh the patient, and transport him or her to the operating room where we would assist with or perform the operation. Ah, those were the days. It was like a Barnum and Bailey version of a medical center.

One night, one of my fellow residents and I were providing post-operative ICU care to a patient who had had cardiac surgery. The patient suddenly started to bleed profusely. Unlike protocols today, which have blood products ready to go, we didn't have any fresh blood on hand. So I, as the senior resident, and Alan Birch, a superstar junior resident, rushed down to the blood bank to give a unit of our own blood for the patient! As we were sitting there with the IV tubing in our arms, we got a call notifying us that there was a cardiac arrest in the ICU.

Like maniacs, we pulled out our IVs, jumped off the cots, and started to run up one level to the ICU. Alan, lightheaded after giving a unit of blood, fainted and fell to the floor. Looking down at him semi-conscious, I said, "Alan, that's okay. You can stay down here. I'm going upstairs." This Keystone Cops kind of rushing around would never happen today in a major or even minor teaching hospital. But the entire event was symbolic of what residents did in those days: everything!

It was all great training for us. Even though we at first were assistant residents—the lowest of the low—we were a band of brothers and sisters and we supported one another. Most of the staff did also.

There was, however, one chief resident superior to me who was a real tyrant. He took great pleasure in disciplining, actually torturing his junior residents. In one case he stressed out a junior resident so much that the poor guy had a gastrointestinal bleed! And this chief resident took some apparent satisfaction in knowing that he was the tough guy who caused it! I was the total opposite in temperament, certainly not a tyrant, then or ever. I may have been tough, but I never wanted to hurt any of my colleagues.

Throughout this period, Dr. Moore had an enormous influence over our lives. Like all great mentors, he established a close relationship with his residents, and treated us with respect even as subordinates. His example would inspire me to do everything I could years later to mentor and pass on my knowledge, a subject to be covered in Chapter 8.

Another legendary figure at the hospital was plastic surgeon Joseph Murray, who ran the Brigham's early and successful human kidney transplant program. It had started auspiciously with identical twin transplants in 1954. For his great path-breaking achievements, Dr. Murray was awarded the 1990 Nobel Prize in Medicine. His pioneering work led to the possibility of other human organ transplants. Murray was not only a brilliant surgeon, but a very down-to-earth, regular kind of guy who regarded residents as colleagues and friends rather than faceless subordinates.

When I first got to the Brigham as a junior resident, Dr. Murray invited all the staff to his house for a party. We had a softball game in which I was pitching. I managed to strike out Dr. Moore two times running, not due to my great athletic ability but because he was constantly swinging and missing! I felt badly, figuring this wouldn't help my future career. But it was all in fun and had no detrimental effect. Joe Murray's hospitality that day typified the good relationships that existed between house and attending staffs, one that I would strive to emulate when I headed up my own service.

Throughout my career, I was meticulous, cool, and calm in the operating room, only demanding in the sense that I wanted everything done in the best way possible. As any surgeon would, I felt it was critical to be in control of things, including my own temper. If I got angry, it was usually because of an administrative error, but even then, I always held myself in check and never reverted to an expression of nastiness. There are enough prima donnas who lose emotional control from time to time.

CHAPTER TWO

SEASONED IN THE ARMY, LAUNCHED INTO THE LAB

F ive years after my internship began, I finished the senior residency at the Brigham, making me board eligible in general surgery. But I was still relatively inexperienced, having performed few major operations—and none of them without supervision.

By this point, you might expect that I was coming out of my shell. But I was still rather shy and somewhat insecure, aware that I was merely a subordinate with a lot to learn. We just did what we were told during those residency years. There were very few times I would proactively show initiative, because I was concerned that it would boomerang.

But now it was time to enter into a new stage of life as I fulfilled my military obligation. I volunteered to be stationed anywhere the army wanted, even in then undesirable Korea. But I fortuitously ended up at Fort Carson, a large army hospital near Colorado Springs that also served the Air Force Academy population.

Looking back, I'd say that the army was a game-changer for me. I was suddenly a *captain* in the US Army Medical Corps, chief of surgery at a large, fully staffed hospital, charged with all the responsibility of performing major operations with no supervision. It was like being thrown into the deep end of the pool.

Due to my youth and relative inexperience surgically speaking, I did not immediately gain the confidence of the hospital commander, a grisly old army colonel who scrutinized my every move. I definitely felt insecure as the new and relatively inexperienced guy on staff. So I worked my butt off day and night, taking excellent care of my patients, many of them elderly army dependents with complex conditions. I was also charged with taking care of the families of the generals and senior officers. Working as hard as I did, and being so attentive to patients, my superiors rapidly interpreted my conscientiousness as competence. And in truth I was getting better and better, with most of my patients recovering well.

One great advantage of working at an army hospital is that you get to do an abundant number of operations, far more than I could ever do at the Brigham. They were mostly routine cases like hernias, gallbladders, radical mastectomies, and gastrectomies. As time passed and my surgical cases produced positive outcomes, I ultimately gained the confidence of my hospital commander, which further bolstered my self-assurance. I knew then that I would be a good surgeon and could do it successfully on my own.

Thereafter, I was allowed to take care of all sorts of complex surgical procedures rather than referring them out to Fitzsimons Army Medical Center, which was a major teaching center in Denver. I found myself doing major pediatric operations, such as those treating an imperforate anus and tracheoesophageal fistula. In fact, I became the pediatric surgery consultant for the entire Fifth Army area, and was referred complex pediatric surgical problems from a five-state area.

Why? Because previously, as part of my Brigham residency, I had spent two months as a junior resident at Boston Children's Hospital where I worked under Dr. Robert Gross, the leading pediatric surgeon of the day. I had read his landmark book *Abdominal Surgery of Infancy and Childhood*, a classic in the surgical literature. I had studied all his descriptions of procedures in that book, and was able to perform some of them with good outcomes. This niche allowed me to get referrals for complex pediatric surgical operations.

During this period, whereas most young doctors were anti-military, I was the exact opposite for all the reasons described earlier. I was relatively conservative, whereas most of the young doctors—then as today—were relatively left-wing. As a result, even though I was the senior surgeon, I volunteered for many unpleasant and sometimes dangerous assignments that many of the other young army doctors would not do. These maneuvers included being part of a rescue team, searching by helicopter in the Colorado mountains for lost soldiers. I also volunteered to serve on the aircraft accident investigating board, a thankless task with reams of paperwork to fill out. I even took lessons and learned how to fly from one of my colleagues on the board.

During this period, I gained a high security clearance, granted to very few, which enabled me to become the support physician and surgeon to highly secretive CIA missions. One of these required the training of foreign national soldiers at Camp Hale, an old army base hidden deep in the Rocky Mountains of Colorado. I had to provide all sorts of care to these foreign soldiers, who were being trained for some sort of insurrection in Asia.

As time passed, I became friendly with the CIA agents who were shepherding the various missions and couldn't help but learn some of the details. Oftentimes the soldiers had sustained serious illnesses or injuries and required immediate hospitalization. These patients would be brought into our hospital in great secrecy in the dead of night. There, just a single corpsman with high security clearance and I had to provide all the patient care without consultation from any specialist. The pressure on us to succeed was tremendous.

One particularly challenging foreign national had a depressed skull fracture of the frontal bone with cerebrospinal fluid leaking out. I was terrified because I had had minimal neurosurgical training. In a flash, I devoured the neurosurgical books I had brought along for emergencies. The text instructed that such injuries into the frontal sinuses required turning a frontal bone flap, something I was totally unable to do! I instead sewed up the soldier's skin wound, gave him high doses of antibiotics, sat up with him for seventy-two hours and prayed!

I couldn't even get nurses or other docs to help because of the secrecy issues. Fortunately, he fully recovered, though he returned to duty with a big crease in his forehead.

Another CIA highlight: A patient was driven into the hospital in the middle of the night with the shades of the CIA SUV drawn down. He was in severe pain with huge strangulated hemorrhoids. I gave him spinal anesthesia and excised the large hemorrhoidal mass. That took care of his hemorrhoids.

However, I had to send the specimen (which looked like a tumor) to the pathologist in order to rule out cancer. My CIA minders would not allow me to put the patient's oriental name on the pathology slip—so I put down my own name! That caused quite a stir with the other doctors in the hospital. "What are you doing with these big hemorrhoids, and who took them off for you?"

On another occasion at Fort Carson, I even got an air force commendation medal for treating a general's son who had sustained hundreds of black gun powder tattoos on his face after a firecracker exploded just in front of him. After many unsuccessful attempts with various methods, including the use of dental drill bits to remove the punctate tattoos embedded in the deeper dermal layers of the skin, I was able to devise a method for removing them by elevating the pin-head sized tattoos with a fine subcuticular needle and shaving off dermis with a blade. The elevating needle provided access to the gun powder in the dermis, but more importantly it controlled bleeding so one could see the extent of the tattoos. The result was complete removal with no scarring. I even published a short paper on the technique, my first ever article.

Overall, I have to say that being thrust into the atmosphere of espionage was exciting to me. I was totally committed to the CIA portion of my duties, enjoying all the cloak and dagger stuff. Most of the time the soldier-patients were young and bounced back quickly, so I was lucky that the outcomes were uniformly good.

As I look back on it now, the army was a hugely maturing experience, giving me seniority as chief surgeon and immense independent experience with patients, much more than I had gotten during my Brigham residency. I even considered staying in the service as a career surgeon and working with the CIA.

But at the end of my two-year stint in the army as a lowly captain, I was superseded by a journeyman lieutenant colonel—a regular army surgeon who demeaned me by putting me on dispensary duty. However, I managed to fulfill this duty quickly in the early morning so I could return to the hospital to perform my scheduled operations without interruption. But when my two years were up, he made it an easy decision to leave the military. I felt fortunate to have served and was now ready to return to the Brigham, where I had been chosen as the chief resident under the renowned Dr. Moore.

As I mentioned, you were treated like a king in your chief resident year, and I guess I enjoyed it as much as any resident could. In my case, Dr. Moore might have started to believe that I was actually getting a little too big for my britches, having had so much surgical experience in the army. He could see that I had returned from Colorado much more confident than I had ever been before.

I admit to organizing, as chief resident, a memorable but drunken Christmas party for one and all. It was a booming success that got a little out of control with a few disheveled staff members passed out in the hallways! From that point on, Dr. Moore banned such parties. My social directorship was over. Oh well.

Like all chief residents at the Brigham, I had been required to spend a year or more of research in the surgical laboratories at Harvard Medical School. Usually this research experience was undertaken before one's chief residency. However, because of my army obligation, it didn't work that way for me. So after completing my chief residency in 1962—making me king for a year—I then launched into my research year as an Arthur Tracy Cabot fellow, working with both Dr. Murray and Dr. Moore in skin and liver transplantation, and the new field of immunosuppression or preventing transplant rejection.

During this period, I also managed to publish several research and clinical articles. All of this combined was very impactful, opening my eyes to the benefits and challenges of an academic career. I had always enjoyed teaching medical students and residents, so this was merely an extension of my growing interest in being not only a surgeon but a teacher and researcher as well.

Being chief resident was an incredibly maturing experience, just as the army had been. I liked all my newfound responsibilities, and the hard work of it all totally agreed with me. In fact, I enjoyed working at the Brigham so much that I wanted to stay on there. But it was then a small hospital and there was no job for me in 1963. Or at least I wasn't offered one.

At this point, with a love for both surgery and research, I remained unsure as to whether I ought to pursue an academic or private practice career. I got a very good private practice offer in White Plains, New York, with a senior general surgeon who had a thriving practice. But I decided that I should remain in the academic sphere.

I accepted a job in the Cornell division at Bellevue Hospital. Unlike the current Bellevue, which has state-of-the-art equipment housed in a modern building serving a wide range of patients, Bellevue back then was an archaic institution serving disadvantaged indigent patients, with big general wards and no private rooms, nothing like what I had been used to at the Brigham.

The basement of the hospital, where I had my little animal laboratory, was right out of a Dickens novel. There I was in a white coat, attempting to concentrate on my work. Meanwhile, I was surrounded by orderlies and maintenance men who were running crap games and smoking drugs. The cards and the dice were flying down there in the environs of hell. No doubt, other nefarious activities were also afoot.

As I could quickly see, ours was the poor sister of the three divisions at Bellevue, with the New York University and Columbia divisions being far better supported and maintained. In fact, because clinical equipment on the Bellevue wards and operating rooms were so limited and primitive for the day, I admit that I would occasionally "transfer" supplies to our wards and animal laboratory from the better-stocked New York Hospital-Cornell, where I had staff privileges.

All in all, despite the anything but glamorous conditions at Bellevue, it was an amazing place to be and especially good for me. Most notably, it gave me a platform and the opportunity to obtain a National Institutes of Health (NIH) grant, which funded my research on artificial oxygenation by venovenous bypass, the precursor of today's ECMO or extracorporeal membrane oxygenation, now an established treatment for severe acute respiratory failure.

While at Bellevue-Cornell, I was also nominated for a prestigious Markle Scholarship—awarded to the most promising young academic scholars from all specialties at all medical schools in the United States. Out of a field of ninety nominees, twenty-five were awarded the sought-after scholarship, and I was fortunate enough to be one of them. In those days, this was a very big deal for an aspiring junior academic surgeon, as it led to additional research dollars and the promise of an eventual leadership position.

While I liked doing the research, and was honored by this award, my position at Bellevue wasn't a good one from an operating surgery point of view. I wanted to do surgery at the level I was accustomed to at the Brigham and in the army. But since it was an entirely resident-run service, I didn't get to do many cases at all. I felt an emptiness at Bellevue without that level of challenge. And though I had staff privileges at New York Hospital, I wasn't able to develop a substantial practice of my own there. Yes, I was doing well academically, but I felt clinically unfulfilled and held back from my true potential.

Then, as fate would have it, one day I picked up the *New York Times* and read that Cornell was withdrawing from its division at Bellevue. My position was thus eliminated through no fault of my own. Suddenly I was out of a job. Making it even more jolting was that I had had to learn about my dismissal in the newspaper rather than from my Cornell superiors. It was pretty disappointing.

However, it is at pivotal moments like these, when a setback is upon you, that you are most likely to gain something even better.

It's amazing how the pathways of a career can occur by accident, how losing one position leads to a lifelong association with a much better job.

That's what happened to me. It wasn't long before I had lots of job offers around the country, largely due to my Brigham training and my NIH and Markle grants. As I considered my options, as always, I wanted to stay in New York. For that reason, I accepted a full-time academic job at Montefiore Medical Center in the Bronx. This job came to me as the result of an offer from Dr. Marvin Gliedman, a friend and fellow Markle scholar, who had just accepted the position as chief of surgery at Montefiore. He wanted me on his team.

My role was to head up a new kidney transplant program and to do general and vascular surgery, both on ward patients and on my own private patients. Not unlike Bellevue, Montefiore was an old institution. Built in 1913, the hospital itself was a run-down physical plant located in a declining and violent inner-city Bronx neighborhood. But it was the primary teaching hospital for Albert Einstein College of Medicine, from which I received my appointment as an associate professor. That sounded good to me.

Like Bellevue, Montefiore served a largely indigent minority population. But it was a private hospital, which had some advantages, and I was able to develop a substantial practice and perform challenging operations on my own patients. I was also able to transfer my Markle scholarship and NIH grants, so I took my laboratory staff with me, allowing my research to continue and grow. It was a definite step up.

My salary at Bellevue-Cornell had been $18,000 per year. Marv Gliedman offered me $30,000. Admittedly, my game plan was to stay at Montefiore for a relatively short time and then move on to a more prestigious academic institution. But that never happened. I would spend most of the rest of my professional career at Montefiore. One major incentive was the complete autonomy I had when it came to directing my own research and surgical work, in addition to controlling some research dollars beyond my grants.

No longer stuck in the dingy basement of Bellevue, I now had expanded laboratory space of my own. I was also able to increase my NIH and other grant support so I could hire a research staff of three trained technicians and a nurse. Moreover, I was able to recruit individuals from other specialties to collaborate in our research. The increase in grants and scientific collaborators facilitated the expansion of my research with an emphasis on lung transplantation—which at that time was the poor sister of the organ transplantation world.

Why was that? Because its clinical application presented what appeared to be unsolvable problems. I was determined to change all that, to establish and eventually turn our hospital's clinical lung transplant service into the preeminent program in the world. It was also at this time that I started a successful kidney transplant program, for which I had unique training at the Brigham.

My decision to balance research and academic work with active surgical practice had a major negative impact on my financial prospects for years to come. In the late sixties, seventies, and eighties, I could have made a fortune in private practice with my background and skills. That was the financial heyday for surgeons in private practice, particularly those doing complex procedures like the ones I did. Many top surgeons had stratospheric incomes in the $2 million range. But I was committed to an academic career and to running my own research program. I wanted to do something that mattered, that made a difference, and that really changed the way medicine was applied to patients. And because my family wasn't poor, I had the resources to supplement my base salary of $30,000 to $100,000 as the years went by. I therefore reconciled myself to trading optimum income for a sense of contribution.

And yet, looking back, I feel like I was exploited at Montefiore. In the 1980s, I would bill and collect more than $2 million for my services. This revenue would go into the department of surgery to support other full-time surgeons who weren't collecting as much. I put aside this inequity, and accepted the monetary situation with the conviction that I was doing the right thing for me. After all, I was running my own impactful research program—one that could hopefully change the medical world. That's what was most meaningful.

So I put much of my focus into research, starting with my passionate commitment to the field of lung transplantation. Here's how it went.

CHAPTER THREE

BREATH IN, BREATH OUT: INNOVATIONS IN LUNG TRANSPLANTATION[1]

A lung equals life.

Pure and simple, the capacity to breathe in and out comprises the essence of existence. At the moment of birth, when a newborn is stimulated to take its first breath, the cycle of life begins. And then it's one breath at a time, in and out, for a lifetime. The movement of the lung upon inhalation provides precious oxygen from the atmosphere for the bloodstream while exhalation rids the body of carbon dioxide. It is a miraculous and automatic reflex.

As physicians, we want those breaths to continue for decades

---

1   The end of this chapter also contains remarks about the definition of death and brain death as they relate to organ transplant donation.

with no interruption. While we can live without an appendix, a spleen, a gallbladder, or a kidney, there is no life without our irreplaceable lungs. In fact, should you lose your lung function for even a few minutes, you're dead.

Breath in, breath out, that's what it's all about.

Breathing is so automatic that it is easy to forget about it altogether until you're having trouble doing it. As we all know, our lungs can get strained, worn out, or diseased through any number of maladies—from emphysema to pneumonia, chronic obstructive pulmonary disease (COPD), cancer, pulmonary hypertension, and beyond.

Enter the reality of lung replacement, a subject that intrigued and fascinated me from the moment I arrived at Montefiore in 1967.

The legendary Dr. Thomas Starzl had pioneered liver transplant surgery in the 1960s, performing the world's first successful liver transplant in 1967. Meanwhile, Dr. Norman Shumway did the same for hearts, performing the first adult heart transplant in the US in 1968, followed by more than a hundred transplants worldwide the same year. Both Starzl and Shumway, who were also my friends, were the superstars of transplantation and research in their particular fields.

Then there was the lung. Going back, the history of lung transplants began with several attempts that were unsuccessful due to transplant rejection. Animal experimentation by various pioneers, including Vladimir Demikhov and Henry Metras during the 1940s and 1950s, first demonstrated that the procedure was technically feasible. James Hardy of the University of Mississippi performed the first human lung transplant in 1963. Following a single-lung transplantation, the patient, identified later as convicted murderer John Richard Russell, survived for eighteen days. From 1963 to 1978, multiple attempts at lung transplantation failed because of rejection and problems with anastomotic bronchial healing. It was only after the development of immunosuppressive drugs such as Imuran (aza-thioprine) and cyclosporin that lungs could be transplanted with a reasonable chance of patient recovery.

From the start, however, I was a pioneer in the field of lung transplantation, conducting key research and clinical studies. In 1972, for example, we transplanted a single right lung into a patient with end-stage emphysema, requiring continuous ventilatory support via a tracheostomy. But after the groundbreaking procedure, which showed that a single transplanted lung could provide total pulmonary function and carry the bulk of the cardiac output, the patient came off the ventilator and improved dramatically. He was able to have his tracheostomy closed, and he could walk around and talk normally for the first time in many years—clearly a dramatic success (see the *Lancet* article in the Appendix).

However, since the patient had been transplanted in the pre-cyclosporin era, he experienced frequent bouts of rejection, which were resolved with large doses of corticosteroids. Amazingly, he lived for six months largely on the function of his transplanted lung. This was an incredible feat.[2]

This achievement certainly paved the way for the first more long-lasting heart-lung transplants performed by Dr. Bruce Reitz of Stanford University in 1981 on a woman who had idiopathic pulmonary hypertension. Two years later came the first long-term surviving single-lung transplant performed by Dr. Joel Cooper in Toronto. (Cooper would use many of the techniques I had developed.)

---

2   A description of this case and the experimental work on which it was based was presented at the American Surgical Association in 1973 and was published in *Annals of Surgery*. This case is also described in a 1972 *Lancet* article, which is reprinted in the Appendix.

My involvement in lung transplantation began in the spring of 1967 when I started my new multi-faceted position at Montefiore as an attending surgeon, researcher, and head of a new kidney transplant program, one of only two in New York City at the time.

By 1967, kidney transplantation was already well established in a number of medical centers. Beginning in 1964, with the routine use of immunosuppressive medication to prevent and treat rejection, the kidney was the easiest organ to transplant: tissue typing was proving helpful; the organ was relatively easy to remove and implant; live donors could be used without difficulty since they could give up one of their two kidneys; and in the event of failure, kidney dialysis was available from the 1940s onward.

The prevailing wisdom in the late sixties was that single-lung transplantation in patients with pulmonary hypertension (a condition in which blood vessels in the lungs are narrowed, blocked, or destroyed) was basically doomed to fail. It was thought that there would always be the insurmountable issue of excessive increased vascular resistance in any transplanted lung due to its obligatory denervation. Such high transplant vascular resistance coupled with the high resistance in the patient's remaining lung would pose an intolerable strain on the heart and render single-lung transplantation impossible, since almost all patients needing a lung transplant had high resistance in their own remaining lung. Moreover, as I've said, lung transplantation had always been the poor sister of heart, liver, and kidney transplants, procedures that had already been performed successfully in patients.

I wanted a new challenge. So in 1967 I had the idea that I should try to overcome the problems that prevented lung transplantation in patients from being successful. There were several reasons behind my idea. Lung transplantation posed unique problems. It offered the opportunity to tread new ground. The lung was a vital organ connected to the circulation with large blood vessels. So it could be transplanted surgically. And if lungs could be transplanted successfully in patients, it would save lives and be worthy of an equally robust transplantation program as hearts, livers, and kidneys.

Despite the obstacles to success, many of which had been identified by prior researchers, I felt that I could tackle and hopefully overcome many of these obstacles. Being young and ambitious, I was determined to make progress that would make lung transplantation feasible as a treatment for patients with end-stage lung disease. In fact, pursuing this path was to become my way of distinguishing myself from those who had come before. Thus began a fifteen-year quest at Montefiore to solve the major challenges that prevented lung transplantation from being a practical treatment.

To begin the journey, the equipment and technician team that I brought from Bellevue to Montefiore was easily adapted from research in extracorporeal assisted oxygenation by venovenous bypass to research in lung transplantation.

To fund my lung transplant research program, I used my existing NIH and Markle grants. We started with animal research, which included multiple experiments studying transplant physiology, preservation, and rejection and its prevention. During the initial experiments, we studied single-lung transplants in dogs. Our goal was to have these single-lung transplants provide total pulmonary function for the animals.

Although I first performed all the technically demanding animal transplants myself, I was soon able to train my two young technicians (with no medical training or experience) to perform the complex animal operations with almost as much skill and finesse as I could. How? Because they did these procedures daily and took on more and more of the responsibility as I was forced to be away for other clinical duties. This gave me enough time to develop a busy surgical practice, which was, of course, a major role for me at Montefiore.

My clinical focus at first was in the areas of vascular, transplant, thoracic, and general surgery for all of which I had been well trained. But gradually my practice involved almost exclusively vascular and transplant patients. Vascular surgery patients with aortic and arterial disease interested me the most. The operations were complex and technically demanding with a huge payoff: saving the lives and limbs of critically ill patients. Best of all, the field was a fertile one for innovating clinical advances.

Meanwhile, our work on animals in the lab was designed to standardize the transplant procedure and to improve upon what others had done. We began by removing a healthy lung from one animal and putting it right back into the same animal (a so-called autograft) eliminating the issue of immunological rejection. Then we occluded the pulmonary artery to the opposite lung so that the transplant would have to provide total pulmonary function to the animal. We also performed lung transplants from one animal to another (an allograft), again occluding the opposite pulmonary artery so the transplant was responsible for the animal's total pulmonary function.

That's where the roadblock occurred. Others had attempted this procedure, but the animals had uniformly died because the vascular resistance in the denervated and transplanted lung was too high for their hearts to tolerate. However, we made the original observation that forcing all the cardiac output through the transplanted lung caused the main (pulmonary) artery to the transplanted lung to dilate substantially. This created a narrowing at the sewn anastomosis (junction) where the transplant pulmonary artery was reconnected to the recipient's pulmonary artery. This narrowing combined with the high blood flow produced a large pressure gradient at the anastomosis and a fatal strain on the heart. When we eliminated this flow-induced narrowing by performing a distensible anastomosis (a connection made surgically between adjacent blood vessels), no pressure gradient occurred when the opposite pulmonary was occluded! The high vascular resistance in the transplant was eliminated and all the animals survived! The transplanted lung that had formerly appeared to demonstrate high vascular resistance no longer did, so the single-lung transplant could provide total lung function for the animal.

This was a potential game-changer for clinical single lung transplantation. Almost all the patients needing a transplant had significant high vascular resistance in their remaining lung. Therefore, the transplanted lung would have to carry most of the cardiac output without straining the patient's heart. Now we knew how to facilitate that.

I was incredibly excited because we had demonstrated that a single-lung transplant could sustain the entire animal if the pulmonary artery anastomosis was made distensible—both with autografts and allografts. Various aspects of this key topic were published in 1969 in the prestigious journal *Science* as well as in various surgical journals.[3]

---

3   Veith FJ, Richards K, "Mechanism and prevention of fixed high vascular resistance in autografted and allografted lungs," *Science* 1969; 164: 699–700.

Remember, this was in 1969 when no one was doing heart-lung transplants or double-lung transplants. Thus, this breakthrough made successful clinical lung transplants feasible.

As time passed, we addressed another key problem with lung transplantation, which was the challenge of healing at the bronchial anastomosis, the main airway of the transplant, which had always been the most vulnerable site for post-operative breakdown and leakage leading to failure. This was almost as big a problem to solve as the apparent high vascular resistance. Both were major obstacles to successful single-lung transplantation, even if rejection could be controlled and prevented.

To solve this bronchial healing problem, we developed an intus-suscepting bronchial anastomotic technique in which the transplant bronchus was telescoped within the host bronchus to prevent leakage. This assured dependable healing of that critical juncture of the transplant. Technical aspects of these important advances were published in 1970 in the widely read journal *Annals of Surgery*.[4]

We also conducted multiple studies on the nature of rejection in lung transplants, though rejection remained a substantial obstacle until the drug cyclosporin came along a decade later, in 1978.

Despite all these advances, our pioneering work in the late sixties and seventies was critically questioned by other surgeon-scientists, who continued to believe that transplanted lungs had an intrinsic high vascular resistance because of the obligatory cutting of their nerves. However, our work showing that the high vascular resistance was at the pulmonary artery anastomosis and not in the lung's intrinsic vasculature would be ultimately confirmed.

---

4   Veith FJ, Richards K, "Improved technique for canine lung transplantation, *Annals of Surgery* 1970; 171: 553–558.

Obviously, because we didn't have cyclosporin during the first decade of our research, we also conducted experiments on immunosuppression (to prevent rejection of transplanted lungs) and developed methods to improve the preservation of lungs outside the body—a key element in any organ transplant, as the organ often needed to be transported from one institution to another. All of this multifaceted work continued to be funded by large NIH grants—over $1 million per year over a fourteen-year period. These grants were awarded after we had performed several partly successful human transplants and many experimental lung transplants in animals.

When rejection was controlled, several of our patients showed that their single-lung transplant could provide very adequate total pulmonary function with low vascular resistance, thereby fully confirming in humans our experimental observations. These observations led to continued funding to support our laboratory and experimental research in all areas of lung transplantation. In addition to addressing rejection and the preservation of donor lungs, we studied the long-term physiology of auto-transplanted lungs and even the feasibility of performing lung transplants between closely related but different species (xenografts from foxes to dogs). Our groundbreaking transplantation work was ultimately reproduced by others and the myth of high vascular resistance making lung transplants intrinsically impossible was debunked once and for all.

Let me now tell you about some of the early and most remarkable cases that are still clearly etched in my mind.

Our most successful transplant patient, who I described at the beginning of this chapter, was a fifty-four-year-old man who was entirely ventilator dependent with a tracheostomy, suffering from end-stage emphysema. After the transplant, he improved dramatically and was sustained solely by his transplanted right lung. It was really a dramatic turnaround for him and a huge boost of optimism for our program and lung transplantation in patients.

We reported this success in 1973 at the American Surgical Association meeting and in the accompanying article on single-lung transplantation in experimental and human emphysema.[5] In this article, we proved that a single lung could provide total pulmonary function in both animals with experimental emphysema and in a patient with severe pulmonary hypertension, and we confirmed in a patient our experimental work on how to prevent the alleged high vascular resistance with a simple technical maneuver at the pulmonary artery anastomosis. This was a major accomplishment, particularly in the era of very primitive immunosuppressive drugs.

Another of our first patients was a fifty-five-year-old woman, existing only on a ventilator with a left lung that was non-functional and a right lung compromised by severe emphysema. She improved immediately with a right lung transplant, but died from a poorly healing bronchial anastomosis—prompting us to develop the intussuscepting bronchial anastomotic technique. We did this with a telescoping anastomosis, which assured adequate blood supply to both components of the anastomosis, which in turn enabled secure healing.

---

5   Veith, FJ, et al., "Single lung transplantation in experimental and human emphysema," *Annals of Surgery* 1973; 178(4): 463–476.

Since we were the only group doing clinical lung transplantation, we attracted a lot of good press. For example, another one of our cases in September and October 1982 was a previously healthy twenty-five-year-old man, a gardener, who had contracted paraquat (a weed killer) intoxication, an often-fatal disease that selectively destroyed the lungs.

The patient was flown into New York from Atlanta for treatment. From the moment I looked at him, only able to breathe with the support of a mechanical ventilator, it was clear that he was dying. It was very sad. With the help of the media, we were able to procure rapidly a healthy donor left lung and to transplant it urgently.

We were in the cyclosporin era by this point, and the patient did not reject the lung. In fact, he did well for several weeks. Then he contracted an overwhelming infection in his remaining paraquat-afflicted right lung, so we removed it. His condition improved, and the left lung transplant was working well and providing excellent total pulmonary function. However, the bronchial closure on the side of his removed infected lung failed to heal and leaked. We attempted to fix the leak, but that too failed because of all the anti-rejection corticosteroids the patient was receiving. Sadly, the young man died seven weeks after receiving his transplant.

This was heartbreaking. We had come so close! The young patient's left lung transplant was providing excellent total lung function—just as we had shown it would experimentally. But no matter how great the effort, doctors are never in control of all the variables.

At the end of this saga, we published an article in the *New York State Journal of Medicine* titled "Single Lung Transplantation in Paraquat Intoxication."[6] This landmark case got me and Montefiore

---

6   Kamholz SL, Veith FJ, et al., "Single lung transplantation in paraquat intoxication," *New York State Journal of Medicine* 1984; 84(2): 82–84.

a great deal of positive media coverage, culminating in a complimentary article in *Time* magazine.

I am sure this *Time* article also elicited some unspoken jealousy and hostility—as positive media coverage usually does. As in any medical institution, doctors and researchers are competitive and not always happy for their colleagues. I am fairly certain that our hospital president felt some resentment about the spotlight being on me, as he believed all rewards should have gone to him. More on colleague relations later.

In another memorable and disappointing case, I was asked to fly to San Francisco General Hospital to treat a ten-year-old boy who was dying of end-stage lung disease. I told the hospital administrators who invited us that I would only make the trip if the hospital could find a donor of an approximate size match. They assured us they could. So off I went, accompanied by my pulmonary medical colleague, Dr. Spencer Koerner, a frequent collaborator on our experimental and clinical cases.

Once we got on the ground, we were sorely disappointed to learn that the donor lung was a size mismatch much larger than the boy. This would make the surgery challenging. Still, the clock was ticking and the boy was near death and worsening. In our desperation to save this boy's life we felt compelled to use the donor lung. Such lungs were scarce. Sadly, it did not turn out well.

During the operation, though the size of the donor pulmonary artery and bronchus did not match those of the boy, we nevertheless managed to put them together with some innovative adaptations. However, the problem came when we attempted to close the boy's small chest cavity around the much larger lung. The lung was markedly compressed and did not function well. The boy lived for several days after the operation as we attempted maneuvers to make the lung function. But because of the size mismatch and some other issues stemming from how sick the boy was, he sadly died. It was a very upsetting experience for the entire group. We had furiously attempted to save his life. My colleague and I flew back to NYC totally discouraged.

All in all, early lung transplantation was not an easy business. It was technically demanding and emotionally draining. Remember, these were still the pioneering days; today, with a proper-sized donor lung, there is a much better chance that the surgery would have succeeded in saving that young boy. In fact, pediatric lung transplants are fairly common today and often successful. According to the National Heart, Lung, and Blood Institute (NHLBI), the one-year survival rate of single-lung transplants is now nearly 80 percent. The five-year survival rate is more than 50 percent. I like to think that this current success rate is in large part due to our work.

In high-profile cases like ours, with hundreds of articles published on our experimental and clinical work, collegial jealousy was at an all-time high. Indeed, nothing generates jealousy and hostility like positive press.

Some of our hospital administrators as well as doctors demonstrated overt hostility, saying we were using up too many institutional resources. This, of course, was discouraging, but I guess this is the way human nature sometimes works.

To reduce stress on my colleagues and myself, I tried to adopt this concept: What other people think of us shouldn't matter if we believe what we are doing is right and will help patients. But I admit the hostility still bothered me.

As for the top management at Montefiore: At first, I was held in high esteem and protected by the president of Montefiore, Dr. Martin Cherkasky. He was a renowned hospital administrator who, over three decades at Montefiore, built it into a respected teaching and clinical institution. He was a true supporter of mine because of my research and leadership efforts and my ability to get NIH grants and other funding.

After his retirement, a subsequent hospital president liked me and often turned to me for advice. As time passed, however, for various reasons, things did not go so well. So I was held in less favor by him and his staff of subservient administrators. He really preferred yes-men around him to someone like me who was outspoken and often went against the grain. Yet despite this tension, my position in the hospital remained secure because of my grants and the large number of patients my vascular surgery service brought into the hospital.

Over a period of fifteen years, based on our research and technical mastery of new techniques, we performed seven clinical lung transplants on desperately sick, dying patients.

You might ask why didn't we do more lung transplants on patients. The answer is simple: we were always hampered by a shortage of suitable donor lungs. Tragically, most patients who needed a lung transplant died while waiting.

In many cases, potential donors lingered until brain death was established. Because of this delay, with mechanical ventilation via endotracheal tubes, they often developed pneumonia, which made their lungs unacceptable as a transplant. Also, unlike kidneys or hearts, size match was a crucial factor for lung transplants. But even when the lungs were viable, sometimes the problem was the unwillingness of competing medical institutions to share suitable lungs—even when they were available!

Montefiore was *not* selfish in that way. For example, when we had a potential heart donor, we would allow another hospital to procure the heart since we weren't performing heart transplants. However, when the roles were reversed and they had a good lung donor, I was surprised that they did not always reciprocate. One has to suppose it was because our hospital might gain stature and publicity by performing a successful lung transplant—but I hope it was for other reasons.

This made clinical lung transplantation very difficult in New York City.

BRAIN DEATH AND THE DEFINITION OF DEATH

Yet another obstacle to finding suitable lungs to transplant was the complex subject of brain death—the irreversible and complete loss of brain function. That's the currently accepted medical and legal definition of death, though certain religious preferences still define death as cessation of heartbeat and respiration. This gives rise to a dilemma.

From our point of view as physicians, transplantation of a viable lung, heart, liver, or kidney is optimal when the brain-dead patient (or donor) is still having his or her respirations, heartbeat, and circulation maintained by a mechanical ventilator. But this can only be accomplished, of course, with the family's permission and when the irreversible death of the donor's brain is established with certainty.

Brain death was an intriguing subject to me. As a lung transplant pioneer and scientist, I strongly advocated for the use of organs from patients who were legally dead on the basis of the irreversible destruction (death) of their brain.

In the mid-1970s I was called to render an expert opinion in a brain death case by a very impressive health care attorney, George Kalkines, then the general counsel of the NYC Health and Hospital System. The case focused on the matter of determining when death occurs and how and when transplanted organs can be used. My position was that brain death equals death, rather than death being defined by the cessation of a heartbeat and respiration.

In this case, controversy arose dramatically on March 4, 1975, when Richard Smith, age twenty-seven, was admitted to the neurological service at Bronx Municipal Hospital Center in a comatose condition, suffering from a gunshot wound to the left temporal area of the brain. The patient was found to be totally unresponsive with no spontaneous respiration or movement. The patient was placed on mechanical respiratory support to assist him during his intensive care unit treatment.

Tests were conducted in accordance with generally accepted medical standards, and it was determined that the patient was neurologically or brain dead on March 5, 1975. The parents of the patient authorized the physicians to remove both kidneys and corneas of the eyes for transplant purposes. Although this patient was a suitable donor and appropriate consents had been obtained from next of kin, the hospital did not proceed to allow removal of organs because of potential legal problems associated with the definition of death, and further by the policy of the chief medical examiner prohibiting removal of organs from homicide victims.

On March 6, the patient, in addition to being dead by neurological criteria (brain death) had cessation of his heartbeat and pulse and was pronounced dead. The organs were not removed, even after his heart had stopped, because of the aforesaid prohibition. As a result, two patients were deprived of kidneys. They had already been identified and were prepared to undergo transplant surgery at Montefiore Medical Center. To me, this was a terrible waste of life-giving organs.

The Smith case typified circumstances that occurred often at that time in all hospitals and which resulted in the unnecessary wastage of organs for transplantation. There was, therefore, great urgency for judicial or legislative resolution of these issues involving the definition of death, brain death and organ donation for transplantation. Because of this Smith Case, Mr. Kalkines sought my opinion about these issues in an attempt to resolve them for the NYC Health and Hospital System better than in the Smith case.

After many discussions with Mr. Kalkines, we became friends and decided that we ought to write definitive articles on brain death and its medical, legal, ethical, and religious ramifications, particularly related to organ transplantation. In this endeavor, we enlisted the collaboration of religious leaders (an Orthodox rabbi and a Catholic priest) and an atheist philosopher. As a result of this meeting of the minds, two widely quoted articles were published in the *Journal of the American Medical Association* (JAMA 1977; 238: 1651 and 1744). These articles were influential in promoting brain death laws in many states that had been without them.

During the writing of these articles, I spent a lot of time visiting with the highest levels of Orthodox rabbinical religious groups in New York City, led by Rabbi Moshe David Tendler, not only a rabbi but a professor of biology at Yeshiva University and an expert in medical ethics. Rabbi Tendler, who co-authored our articles, advocated the theory that complete and irreversible cessation of function of the entire brain renders a person "physiologically decapitated," and is therefore legally dead according to Jewish law. Rabbi Tendler further asserted that once organ donation has been deemed permissible under the given conditions, it is indeed mandatory, falling under the rubric of the legal obligation of Jews to preserve the lives of others. He and I were soul mates in this crusade to save the lives of others by transplanting organs from those who were never to recover.

Rabbi Tendler's support led to acceptance of the brain death concept on a larger scale. Together, we promoted the concept of brain death in our legislature and in other states around the country. To this end, I led the effort in New York State to get a law passed recognizing the legality of brain death. I got Orthodox rabbis and Catholics (who had previously been largely opposed) to collaborate in the effort to get the brain death law passed.

It was a very exciting effort in which we took busloads of people (transplant recipients and their families) to lobby the state legislature. We received a fair amount of favorable press coverage and I got an op-ed titled "Statutory Recognition of Brain Death" published in the *New York Times* on May 20, 1976.

In the op-ed, I indicated the legal jeopardy of physicians who allowed transplant donation after brain death without the protection of a state law that recognized and permitted it: "Should doctors pronounce death based on total irreversible loss of brain function when such pronouncements may be disputed in a judicial proceeding on the basis of the common-law definition that death occurs only when spontaneous respiration and heartbeat cease? Without statutory or case-law recognition of brain death, it is possible that a valid medical declaration of death could be considered illegal and lead to criminal or civil liability on the part of a physician or hospital."

I advocated for a statutory definition of death which would help guarantee the highest standard of medical science. As I concluded: "For these reasons, passage of legislation defining death and recognizing brain death has gained widespread support from prestigious representatives of the Roman Catholic, Jewish, and Protestant faiths as well as from the organizations representing the legal profession and the medical profession in New York State.

"It is clear that passage of such timely legislation is urgently needed to modernize the law in keeping with current advances in medical technology and practice and to make certain that the diagnosis of death will be made with the greatest possible care."

Although I had devoted a huge amount of my time to lung transplantation, there came a point when I finally decided to transition past it. Yes, our work had led to trailblazing research and the clinical successes of our team and others, as well as the publication of multiple scientific articles and the awarding of large NIH grants. But even in the face of all these herculean efforts, our work led to relatively few lung transplant patients in New York City for some of the reasons already mentioned.

I had the feeling at the time in NYC that human lung transplantation was not an area where I could really grow clinically, because the cases were so few and far between and lung donors were so limited. I felt that I should maintain and advance my surgical skills with patients. I also believed that I should focus on one subspecialty of general surgery, rather than the entire spectrum, and that I should become expert in that one area. The area that appealed to me most was vascular surgery. It was technically demanding and a relatively new area that could lend itself to further research and advances if one could develop innovative techniques or approaches.

I therefore elected to focus a major part of my clinical attention on the care of vascular disease patients and related innovative research in vascular surgery, a niche that I was trained for and one that would provide me with a large number of operative cases.

I had been named chief of vascular surgery at Montefiore Medical Center and Albert Einstein College of Medicine in 1971, but had split my efforts between lung transplantation and clinical vascular surgery until 1986. From that point onward I decided that my lung transplantation efforts should end so that I could devote my full attention to vascular surgery and research related to it. It was my next mountain to climb

CHAPTER FOUR

THE ART OF LIMB SALVAGE

Among all operations performed on patients, there are few that are as psychologically devastating as a major limb amputation. What could be more traumatic than the severance of a body part? Whether it's an above- or below-the-knee amputation, the removal of an arm, or even a lesser amputation, the patient is losing a part of themselves.

Whether due to a war wound, an accident, a malignancy, or ischemic gangrene the removal of a limb can be a terrifying shock and disabling. It will also tremendously impact a patient's self-image, their career, and their relationships. In fact, according to multiple studies, a substantial proportion of amputees have alarming signs of depression, suicidal ideation, and post-traumatic stress disorder (PTSD).

Thirty percent of amputees are troubled by severe depression due to decreased self-esteem, distorted body image, increased dependency on others, and social isolation. Cosmetic appearance also plays a huge role in the psychological impact of limb removal; a person's picture of themselves is profoundly disrupted when a limb is amputated. There is, no doubt, a need to form a liaison between surgical treatment providers and psychiatrists and psychologists to manage psychiatric comorbidity in amputees.

However, the best thing is to prevent a major amputation in the first place, if it can be done without costing a patient's life. Amputations, including the most common ones of the lower limb, have been performed for centuries, and they are still being done in large numbers around the world—mostly because of poor arterial circulation.

The first known reports of amputations originate from ancient ruins in Egypt, where primitive prosthetic toes were found in the tombs of the Pharaohs. In Europe, during the period of ancient Greece and Rome, various examples of amputations were described on amphorae and mosaics. True advances in amputation and prosthetic techniques took place during the Renaissance and the centuries that followed. And the greatest developments in limb amputation techniques and prosthetic methods began in the twentieth century.

No matter what the era, when amputation is required, the physician must take swift action to save a life, removing all damaged tissue while leaving behind as much healthy functioning tissue as possible.

Age makes a great difference in how people react and recover from such procedures. For example, the removal of a limb in an elderly sick patient with arteriosclerosis (due mainly to poor arterial blood supply or blocked arteries) can be serious, leading to severe disability or death. Even when things go well, the road to recovery and rehabilitation isn't an easy one.

A few of the aged with lower limb amputations (i.e., below-the-knee removals) may be able to walk limited distances. But rarely do they ambulate well with an artificial limb. If it's a more extreme above-the-knee amputation, rehabilitation and walking is even more problematic in the elderly. In contrast, the same amputations in a young healthy person (followed by fitting the patient with a modern prosthesis) can lead to successful rehabilitation, and to normal physical mobility.

No matter what the age, a positive attitude and perseverance are often the elixirs to healing and good ambulatory function. Indeed, many younger patients, especially soldiers, adapt well with optimism and gratitude. They find relief in the elimination of pain and find positive meaning in the procedure. They can develop improved coping abilities, an enhanced spiritual life, and can even inspire others with their resilience and ability to live life to the fullest. However, saving the limb, if possible, is always preferable to a major amputation

One of the most compelling events in my career was the case of tennis champion Carol Ligotino, a then-sixteen-year-old Bronx, New York, native who was brutally attacked by a rapist in 1981.

Before that horrible night, the strong and athletic high school junior was already nationally recognized as an up-and-coming tennis superstar, ranked twentieth in the world and mentored by the likes of Billy Jean King and Martina Navratilova. But on December 22 her life took a tragic turn.

While walking home from a subway station, Carol was accosted and dragged into a park at knifepoint by an attacker intending to rape her. She resisted. He then viciously stabbed her in the right side of her chest. When he attempted to stab her chest a second time, the blonde-haired teenager thrust her right leg into the knife's path, and it plunged between both bones of her leg, severing all three of its arteries just below the knee.

The despicable attacker fled and left Carol on the ground bleeding. However, she managed to stagger out of the park onto a street below an elevated subway. She then lay in the dark, rain-soaked street unable to move. Several passing cars refused to even stop; they swerved around her prostrate form.

Because of her chest injury and the bleeding, she could have easily died there in the street. However, a gypsy cab driver (recently released from jail for murder) spotted Carol, put her in his car, and brought her to the now-defunct Pelham Bay General Hospital. He was the true hero of the night.

The attending surgeon at Pelham Bay inserted a chest tube and saved Carol from a tension pneumothorax. However, he was considering the need to amputate her right leg, which was ischemic and bleeding profusely below the knee.

Thankfully, Carol's mother knew of our limb salvage work at Montefiore from some of the public recognition we had received. I will soon explain its history. She somehow found my phone number and called me. (I always gave my phone numbers out to patients who asked for it.)

Because I was at our division Christmas party that night, I told Carol's mother to bring Carol to our hospital emergency room at Montefiore and that the vascular surgeon on call would take care of her and call me if necessary. Unfortunately, the vascular surgeon on call that night was not particularly skilled, though he stopped the bleeding and evacuated the hematoma. He also obtained an arteriogram confirming the severance of the three leg arteries, but did nothing more.

The next morning, that surgeon called me quite upset because the girl's right leg was now cadaveric—cold, blue, and paralyzed. He implored me to take over this case because he was worried about being sued, cognizant that Carol was a rising tennis star about to lose her leg.

I agreed to operate on Carol's leg in an effort to save it, recognizing that we might not be successful. Fortunately we were able to do one of the procedures that I had innovated, a popliteal-to-tibial artery bypass from the artery behind the knee to one of the smaller arteries in the lower leg. We had developed this procedure to treat severe foot ischemia by bypassing blocked leg arteries to restore arterial circulation to the lower leg and foot.

One of the great challenges in a young person like Carol was that her leg arteries were tiny, only about 1.5 mm or less in diameter, because they were in spasm. Though she was perilously close to losing her leg, my bypass to her small artery fortunately worked and her leg was saved.

But, as we told Carol's mother, it was not known if Carol would ever regain partial or full use of the leg. Carol bravely told a newspaper reporter at the time: "I'm not thinking of that possibility. I'm strong. This isn't going to stop me. I'm going to stay tough." And we felt that her huge desire to get better might very well impact the results.

Unfortunately, either the initial knife wound or the work of the first surgeon injured Carol's peroneal nerve, which left her with a slight foot drop, an inability to lift the front part of the foot. Although she was ultimately able to walk and run normally again, this condition was a game-changing disability for the aspiring tennis player. No longer could she compete at the highest level. Her burgeoning career in professional tennis was over.

But as often happens in young patients, Carol's energy and natural ebullience eventually returned. She recovered physically quite well, could walk normally, play tennis (and golf, at which she became expert), and went on to lead a very productive life as a mother and successful business owner. In years subsequent to the surgery, we remained good friends. In fact, at one point I played tennis with her and she was still quite amazing—every shot within a foot of the lines. Who knows what she could have accomplished had this event never happened?

As I think back to it now, Carol's story is one of many compelling examples of why I became fascinated with the mission of saving lower limbs in the first place.

In 1971, I was made chief of the vascular surgery division at Montefiore. Back then, the prevailing wisdom of the day was that any surgical attempt to bypass or remove blockages and improve the blood supply to a gangrenous foot or a threatened limb due to hardening of the arteries or arteriosclerosis below the groin was likely to fail. Previous attempts had often resulted in higher levels of amputation above the knee and was therefore not generally considered worthwhile.

So, in the late sixties and early seventies, the standard of care for most patients with ischemic gangrene, ulceration, or severe rest pain was to perform a below-knee amputation and hope that the patient could be rehabilitated with a prosthesis or artificial limb. Several scholarly articles in medical journals supported the concept that reconstructive arterial surgery below the groin when a limb was threatened was risky, did not work well, and often caused more harm than good.

But why hadn't reconstructive arterial procedures to bypass obstructions worked? In my view, it was a blend of factors: some

surgeons followed prevailing opinions and avoided these procedures, or they couldn't perform the procedures well or carefully
enough for them to work. Others didn't have the ability to perform
accurate arteriography, which would show arteries that could be
used as bypass targets—subjects I'll address in a moment.

Also, limb salvage operations, even when attempted, were labor
intensive, could take many hours, and required a meticulous commitment to detail and technical perfection. Doing such procedures
wasn't as cost effective or as time efficient as performing a major
amputation. And to say the unsayable: some surgeons wanted to
perform the easier, more standard vascular procedures, such as
operations on the aorta and carotid arteries, all of which took less
time and effort and were compensated by superior reimbursement
and larger fees.

From my point of view, time and money aside, if we could save
a leg and keep it functional, *and* keep patients out of nursing homes
(which would save a great deal of money too), limb salvage surgery
was well worth it! Yet, as I've stated, it was widely believed that such
limb-saving procedures would not work even if attempted.

But I did not agree with this thinking. I refused to yield to the
defeatist convention about automatic amputation. Just as we had
pioneered in lung transplantation, we now went against the grain
by demonstrating that limb-saving bypasses to even diseased, very
distal arteries could work, and that extensive gangrene of the foot
and heel did *not* require a major amputation. After a successful
bypass, one could debride even extensive gangrene and obtain a
healed foot and a useful extremity.

So, beginning in the early 1970s, I cautiously began doing
reconstructive arterial bypasses for disease below the inguinal
ligament and into the leg below the knee to salvage these limbs

that others thought to be unsalvageable. Much to my delight and somewhat to my surprise, when we performed these infrainguinal bypasses (below the groin) with meticulous vein graft conduits (or prosthetic grafts in patients without good veins), most of these procedures worked.

One contributing factor to our success was that we were using semi-microsurgical techniques and instruments, similar to those we had been using to create arteriovenous fistulas for dialysis patients with end-stage renal disease.

Based upon our early success, we were emboldened to do more and more aggressive and more distal bypass procedures to save limbs that were deemed hopelessly unsalvageable by others. Over the next decade, although others thought we were crazy, we developed and refined effective and unusual techniques for artery bypasses, performing thousands of successful limb salvage procedures in patients with severely threatened limbs. We were able to save over 90 percent of these limbs. Patients were able to walk again and to be cared for at home.

While what we were doing was unique and consistently successful, our commitment to limb salvage, as I said, ran against the grain of then-current vascular surgical thinking. Most others would not or could not perform these limb salvage procedures. Importantly, our over 90 percent success rate included patients who had been unsuccessfully operated on by others, as well as those in whom we had done a bypass that worked for a while and then failed.

Our team was the first to show that redo bypasses were worthwhile as we developed special techniques for performing those redo procedures, including the use of prosthetic bypasses to artery targets above and below the knee, and even to smaller arteries in the leg. (The use of prosthetic bypasses to such tibial arteries remains controversial, although we have continued to show that such procedures are effective when other options are not available—sometimes working effectively for more than five years.)

Gradually, however, other vascular surgeons confirmed the value of our aggressive approach to limb salvage and adopted it— although they sometimes sadly posed as the innovators and rarely gave us credit for pioneering this approach. In fact, many of those who originally treated our work with disdain and skepticism subsequently adopted our techniques. Some even claimed credit for being the original advocates. More on that a bit later in the chapter.

I was not surprised by this collegial jealousy after the reception I first received when I was made chief of vascular surgery in 1971. As a full-time surgeon and researcher in what was then a largely private practice hospital, I was the immediate target of hostility, partly due to what I'll call *town/gown* friction.

At the time, there were eleven mostly private practice general surgeons who dabbled in vascular surgery on my service. Though they were selling themselves as vascular surgeons, they really weren't. After I was made the chief, I found that they were unified in one mission—getting rid of me as the chief.

At first, I tried to be affable and supportive of what they were doing, and limited myself to cases that they didn't want to take on. But that didn't work. To my dismay, I found out that all eleven met on a nightly basis in one of their houses to plan a way to depose me. I found this out when two of them turned on their colleagues, told me about the conspiracy, and offered to join me if I would share my patients and research facility with them. I did so. That defused the conspiracy.

Moreover, even before my innovations in limb salvage surgery were evolving and the findings getting published in first-line journals, I was able to outperform most of the conspirators because I did *only* vascular surgery. This was supplemented by kidney and lung transplant surgery, which was largely vascular surgery from a technical perspective. So I rapidly became better at the specialty—better than those who did it part time.

To appease my opposers, I still referred a large number of private patients to the other surgeons, though I took the most difficult cases, the ones that interested me most. This included the limb salvage cases that would help define my career in vascular surgery.

Ultimately, as pioneers in limb salvage surgery at Montefiore, my team saved thousands of patients from the anguish and disability that occurs after a major lower limb amputation. This early record of success with limb salvage surgery fortuitously opened up an entirely new area within the specialty of vascular surgery, one that thwarted the status quo and established me as an iconoclast and leader within the field.

What was driving me toward specializing in limb salvage in the first place? It was partly out of necessity.

From when I first arrived at Montefiore in 1967 and extending to when I became chief in 1971, I wanted to perform all the standard and popular arterial operations of the day—carotid endarterectomies, aortic aneurysm repairs, and aorto-femoral bypasses. But, to my dismay, there were an inadequate number of elective arterial cases of this sort available to me. These kinds of patients were not exactly pouring through our doors in great numbers, as Montefiore was considered a second-tier hospital amongst the most prestigious institutions in New York City.

In addition, the patients who did exist were sent to older general surgeons with established referral patterns, the so-called old boy's network. This did not include a thirty-five-year-old newcomer like me. But there was no way I was going to feel clinically satisfied with such a paucity of standard vascular surgery cases.

However, I noticed that there *was* a large indigent population in the Bronx, many of them poor elderly patients mostly from the Black and Hispanic communities. These patients, with a high incidence of diabetes, had limbs threatened by ischemic gangrene of the toes or feet, severe ischemic rest pain, or extreme ulceration resulting from arteriosclerotic arterial occlusive disease (blocked arteries). Very few had conditions that were suitable for treatment by large artery aorto-bifemoral bypass.

However, many of them had arterial blockages below the groin, and many more had arterial blockages at multiple levels, including those in the smaller arteries of the leg and foot. Most of these blockages in arteries in the leg and foot were unrecognized. Why? Because other institutions did not obtain adequate arteriograms, the imaging test that uses x-rays and a special contrast agent to image the inside or luminal channel within the little patent arteries below the knee and in the lower leg and foot. But we went the extra mile.

Let me explain why we had such good arteriograms to facilitate limb salvage at Montefiore: When I took over as chief of vascular surgery, all twelve of our vascular surgeons did their own arteriograms or angiograms. They were of mixed or poor quality. I passed a rule that only our interventional radiologist could perform such arteriograms—*all* of them.[7] Why? Because he consistently delivered precise images of the open arteries at every level including

---

7   However, this practice meant that we as surgeons lost our catheter guidewire skills—a decision of mine that later proved to be a mistake as we had to relearn them years later as endovascular treatments exploded.

those in the lower leg and foot. Some of these arteries had not been recognized by other hospitals because their arteriograms were not as good. But we found patent arteries that others didn't even look for because they did not include the lower leg and foot in their arteriograms.

That's why patients started coming to us after being told by vascular surgeons in other hospitals that amputation was their only recourse. We would repeat the arteriogram (we called it getting a "real arteriogram"), see the patent distal arteries, and use them for a bypass target to save the limb! With our excellent distal and complete arteriograms, we were able save 90 to 95 percent of all threatened limbs in patients with and without diabetes.

And if you asked the patient whether or not the time and discomfort of their procedures were worth it, they would laugh. Of course, it was worth saving their leg. Word about our success rate spread, with referrals flooding in from other hospitals—patients hopeful that we'd figure out a way to save their leg. We tried to accommodate everybody. Much to the chagrin of other practitioners, we were often successful when other first-rate institutions like the hospitals of Cornell, NYU, Columbia, and Mount Sinai had failed one or more times.

In short, I had been convinced that most patients with threatened limbs had patent arteries to which a bypass could be constructed so that circulation could be restored to the foot and the limb saved. This premise turned out to be correct and enabled us to save a large number of limbs others thought to be unsalvageable. Most other vascular surgeons did not even look for very distal patent arteries—and as a result, did not find them.

Our success in this area was pivotal for me. I thought to myself, this is a part of a specialty that I could make my own, one that could provide a rich research opportunity and an avenue of service to others. Rather than acquiescing to the automatic standard of a major amputation, I could find better ways to avoid them.

I should say that several pioneers before me had done successful bypasses designed to cure the condition of pain while walking and occasionally for limb salvage. These operations were usually at the aorto-femoral level, requiring an incision in the abdomen, or to arteries in the thigh.

Drs. Michael DeBakey, Emerick Szilagyi, Sterling Edwards, and Jack Wylie performed large numbers of aorto-femoral bypasses. Jean Kunlin was the originator of the reversed vein graft in the thigh. Dr. Szilagyi and John Mannick were advocates for vein bypasses below the groin. However, these were feasible in only a minority of patients with threatened limbs. I was also the one most often regarded as the pioneer in the use of polytetrafluoroethylene (PTFE) prosthetic bypasses below the groin and to arteries below the knee—even those in the lower leg.

But bypasses below the inguinal ligament (groin) and especially those done with prosthetic (Dacron or PTFE [Teflon]) grafts had usually failed. When that happened, the limbs became ischemic and an amputation—often at a higher level—would be required. So, while vein grafts in the thigh were innovated before me in a small percentage of patients, the field of innovative techniques in limb salvage was still wide open.

At Montefiore, I and my group were the first to advocate an aggressive approach to salvaging most threatened lower extremities by performing what turned out to be pioneering bypasses with vein or prosthetic (PTFE) conduits or grafts.

Since most of these patients had complex, multilevel and distal occlusions below the knee, they often required very distal small leg artery bypasses to save their legs. Such conditions with very distal disease and occlusions are particularly common in diabetics and in patients with end-stage kidney disease. Arterial occlusive disease and arteriosclerosis is also aggravated in smokers. We found successful ways to save the limbs of patients in all these higher risk groups of patients.

Ordinarily, in cases with extensive multilevel occlusive disease (when tissue dies as manifest by gangrene or ischemic ulceration), patients were considered inoperable and referred for an amputation. However, with our complete arteriograms, we found that the blood supply could almost always be improved by an arterial bypass with salvage of the threatened limb.

Once we established ourselves as innovators and leaders in limb salvage, the perception of our hospital changed. Though Montefiore was considered by some to be a second-rate hospital (and in many ways it was), having superb arteriography and exceptional limb salvage results made a big difference in our hospital's reputation.

Yet I'd have physicians and researchers coming from England and Europe to the Bronx, to question our results *and* my judgment and to see our techniques. Often they would be convinced, but sometimes they would not, saying these techniques are just too difficult and not possible in their institution. Some even went so far as to say: "We don't get angiograms that show those vessels as being visible and viable targets for a bypass. You're out of your mind. You can't do a bypass to those tiny diseased arteries."

They didn't get it. We weren't out of our minds. We were right, and I and my partners could do a successful bypass to them!

As I demonstrated again and again, we were the first to visualize distal small arteries with great accuracy, find patent target arteries in the lower leg and foot, and thereby perform successful bypasses.

If the first procedure failed, we often re-operated and ultimately got the result we wanted. We were able to save almost all (more than 90 percent) of the threatened limbs that came to us.

I was also very aggressive about debriding foot wounds, believing that older sick patients could walk on even a small remnant of foot better than after a major amputation.

We also challenged the idea that you shouldn't do bypass procedures on patients who were sick with co-morbidities, such as congestive heart failure, lung disease, cancer, or extensive gangrene of the heel. Others considered these patients too risky or unsuitable for bypass procedures. Nonetheless, we persevered, went against the grain again, and found that patients with these conditions could be treated with good results if they received technically perfect surgery, expertly administered anesthesia, and excellent post-operative care, thereby proving old assumptions wrong. And although the operations often were difficult and long, sometimes lasting over six hours, we were able to save most of these legs.

After the first wave of successful limb salvage at Montefiore, we became emboldened and tried to save almost all of the threatened legs aggressively. Over the next ten years, we developed all sorts of techniques for treating threatened limbs. Our success was due to a number of factors: first, as I've stated, we did very careful graft-to-artery micro-anastomoses to the small distal arteries; second, we went the extra mile and re-operated on patients after a procedure failed; and third, we were very aggressive about cleaning up the gangrenous and infected tissue in the foot or heel and getting healed wounds after our bypasses restored good circulation.

A fourth, and very significant addition to this list, I early on embraced endovascular balloon angioplasty and stenting, typically used to eliminate occlusions in the iliac or femoral arteries proximal to more distal disease that needed to be treated by a bypass. (The balloon restores the lumen or blood flow channel to a blocked artery; a stent is a metal framework that can be expanded to maintain the restored arterial lumen.) These minimally invasive procedures eliminated the need, in our fragile limb salvage patients, to do aorto-femoral bypasses, a stressful and morbid open operation conducted through a long incision in the abdomen.

In the late nineteen seventies, we were among the first to use balloon angioplasty to treat occluded artery patients at a time when other vascular surgeons were denying their value. We used this method because it was less invasive, easier, and safer, especially when a patient had complex multilevel occlusive disease, as was the case in most patients with a threatened limb.

Of course, endovascular techniques today are the hottest topic in vascular treatment. The field has exploded, with all doctors preaching in favor of aggressive limb salvage. But it was our team that originally advocated this approach in almost all such patients.

I first learned about the technique of balloon angioplasty when I was president of the New York Cardiovascular Society. In the late nineteen seventies, at a meeting of that society, I had invited a pioneering US radiologist to speak, Dr. Charles Dotter. He was credited with establishing the subspecialty of interventional radiology, the use of medical imaging to guide minimally invasive endovascular or endolumenal tools to restore the central blood flow channel or lumen to obstructed or occluded arteries.

Dr. Dotter, together with his German-born colleague, Dr. Andreas Gruentzig, were pioneers of using small, flexible, plastic tubes or catheters to re-open a severely narrowed or occluded artery in the thigh, a procedure which they called percutaneous transluminal angioplasty (PTA). Gruentzig's contribution was to place a non-compliant balloon on the distal end of a catheter to make the dilating or widening procedure more effective. For these innovations they were nominated for the Nobel Prize in Physiology and Medicine in 1978—although sadly they never received the award.

Over the next decades, PTA, or balloon angioplasty, became the method of choice to effectively treat legions of patients with narrowed or occluded arteries to or in the lower extremity or heart. When the balloon tipped catheter is in place, its inflation opens the central channel or lumen of the artery, so that normal blood flow is restored. But even before the balloons were used, Dotter had introduced tapered catheters that also dilated narrowed or occluded artery lumens. The value and durability of PTA was subsequently enhanced by the addition of stents (expandable metal cages or frameworks) which would hold the dilated arteries open by preventing elastic recoil. Nevertheless, PTAs and stents still sometimes failed because of a process called intimal hyperplasia—the healing proliferative response in a traumatized blood vessel. That process is inhibited by coating the balloon with drugs like Paclitaxel or other agents. This is the state of the art today.

Back in the late seventies, this technique sounded strange to many vascular surgeons with closed minds when they heard his presentation at our New York Cardiovascular Society meeting. They thought Dotter made no sense as he described the process of dilating an arteriosclerotic plaque-filled artery.

"It's like creating a footprint in the snow," he told us. "You compress the plaque, it gets smaller. The artery lumen is increased and flow is re-established."

After hearing that, every other surgeon in the audience said it was nonsense, that it would fail. They dubbed Dotter "Crazy Charlie."

Initially, I was skeptical myself; I thought Dotter's technique probably wouldn't work—but then again maybe it *could*. And if it did, I could see how PTA would be a less invasive method that could greatly benefit our high-risk limb salvage patients, many of them old and sick, not suitable candidates for a major operation like an aorto-femoral operation to bypass occluded or narrowed iliac arteries in the lower abdomen.

With that in mind, I persuaded our interventional radiologist, Dr. Seymour Sprayregen, to travel out to Portland, Oregon, to observe Dr. Dotter as he performed the tapered catheter angioplasties at his hospital. When Sprayregen returned to Montefiore a few weeks later, he reported how effectively this protocol had worked. Once I heard this, I thought we ought to try to do the procedure at Montefiore. We never looked back, becoming one of the first surgical groups to embrace PTAs—first with the tapered catheters of Dotter, then with the balloon catheters of Gruentzig, and, when they became available, the stents of Dr. Julio Palmaz and others.

I would stand in the angiography suite as Dr. Sprayregen performed the tapered catheter angioplasties (at first doing iliac artery angioplasty instead of an aorto-femoral bypass). Once the iliac PTA worked, we could then perform a successful infrainguinal bypass with acceptably good inflow, avoiding the need for a big open abdominal operation.

Our mastery of these combined procedures furthered our leadership position in the area of limb salvage. We were then referred patients with difficult lower-extremity ischemia problems not only from our own tri-state area but from all over, even as far away as India. These were almost always patients with severely threatened legs who had been given up at other hospitals for any attempt at limb salvage. Now they came in abundance to us in the Bronx.

Over and over again, we led the way, performing surgery on patients deemed unsuitable for any kind of limb saving procedure by
everybody else, namely with very distal disease, requiring a bypass
to a very small artery in the distal leg or the foot. We challenged
these contraindications to limb salvage surgery and often succeeded. (At times, even I was shocked that many of these difficult procedures were successful.)

Together with my trainee and then partner, Dr. Enrico Ascher,
we did procedures to save limbs in difficult circumstances—procedures that even we considered impossible. We even attempted
to do arterial bypasses to veins in the foot when no patent target
arteries were present. Dr. Ascher had some limited success with
these procedures. Today, with improved technology for destroy-
ing the valves in veins so blood could flow backwards into arteries
and capillaries, these procedures are being done widely with good
success. Importantly, Dr. Ascher has become a prominent leader in
vascular surgery, largely because of his pioneering efforts in limb
salvage and finding better ways to image arteries with ultrasound.

Of course, we were very interested in widely publishing and
teaching others our techniques. This included presenting our data
and publishing the results in respected first-line medical and surgical
journals. The press and the electronic media also became interested in our work and covered it widely. We did not discourage
this because we felt it would be of value and helpful to patients. After
all, we were doing pioneering work that resulted in overwhelmingly
positive results. Why not talk about it and make other physicians
aware so they could save these threatened limbs too?

Admittedly, the downside of our techniques, which sometimes
required multiple procedures, was that they often required longer
hospital stays. Needless to say, our hospital administrators were

quite displeased by these patients' long lengths of stay (LOSs), which were expensive, as we were only being reimbursed for shorter ones. So we worked to decrease the lengths of stay and were somewhat successful at it.

Our first summary limb salvage publication was in 1981 and described five-year results in 689 patients having various bypass operations and angioplasties.[8] Our second major paper was published in 1990—although we had hundreds of articles on related topics by that time—and it described the patterns of arterial disease we were recognizing and treating, and results in 2,829 patients.

Bypass procedures to heavily calcified arteries (widely considered impossible to treat) were just one example of what we were able to do successfully. These were described in an article with Dr. Ascher as the first author. Use of isolated segments of arteries as a target for a prosthetic bypass was another generally held contraindication that we challenged successfully. And leaving all or part of an infected graft in a patient and getting a healed wound and a salvaged limb was yet another. These procedures (discussed more fully in Chapter 8) were described in several articles first authored by another trainee and colleague, Dr. Keith Calligaro. He has also become a respected leader in vascular surgery.

By doing all this, we challenged the thinking of the day: that you shouldn't perform distal bypass procedures for limb salvage, much less on patients who had serious co-morbidities like cancer or heart failure. Moreover, surgical experts of the day said with great authority that infected arterial grafts had to be surgically removed completely.

---

8   Veith FJ, et al, "Progress in Limb Salvage by Reconstructive Arterial Surgery Combined with New or Improved Adjunctive Procedures," *Annals of Surgery* 1981; 194: 386–399.

At first, I believed the latter too. But when we surgically removed them, the patient would end up losing their leg or their life. I therefore tried leaving them in, and surprisingly, if we debrided the surrounding wound adequately, it often worked—with up to twenty-five years follow-up in one patient. (Dr. Calligaro has published many important journal articles about these procedures. I first described them in an unreferenced book chapter but have never had a first-authored publication on the topic, although I took most of the heat for promoting this against-the-grain technique!) It still remains somewhat controversial, but others have confirmed that such graft-sparing techniques can sometimes work. Obviously, these techniques must be used selectively and judiciously and be implemented with appropriate precautions.

Another of my against-the-grain innovations was originating bypasses for distal arteries at or below the knee, rather than originating them all from the groin, as was the standard of the day. This allowed shorter segments of vein to be used when patients did not have longer segments of vein for a bypass conduit. It yielded good results especially in patients with very distal patent target arteries to bypass to.

Many conditions were considered contraindications to successful limb-saving bypass procedures. Yet we usually found ways to overcome these presumed negatives and perform effective and durable bypasses with successful limb salvage.

All in all, we published over a hundred articles on the subject of lower-extremity and limb salvage surgery (plus numerous chapters in books as well). Yet, despite our proven advances, we were often greeted with much skepticism, even disdain and occasional ridicule, from many of my medical and surgical colleagues. They usually liked me personally, but they didn't always agree with our aggressive approach and its techniques. They also found our results difficult to reproduce and therefore doubted them. Indeed, at regional, national, and international surgical conferences, we were often scoffed at because we were introducing new ideas and techniques—going against the grain of current thinking and practice.

"Why are you doing these lengthy and complex procedures? Isn't it better to just cut the leg off?"

They really thought it was. But we knew it wasn't.

So we had to prove our procedures worked and truly helped patients. I remember that when one of my trainees presented these techniques at a national meeting, the moderator, a prominent vascular surgeon of the day (John Mannick), quipped, "You must work with that crazy guy Veith in the Bronx!" But that kind of skepticism only fueled our resolve.

What particularly irked me was that many doctors doubted our success rates, believing that we were either lying or misguided. We were neither. We were revolutionaries, going against the grain, doing something that other surgeons and researchers hadn't done, succeeding where others had failed. We were scrupulously honest in collecting and reporting our data, and we wanted others to understand what we were able to do, because it was good for patients. It was therefore troubling to have our reports and presentations sometimes so poorly received.

I understood that we would be challenged by others who questioned our innovations. This and other experiences taught me that man can be a very hostile, jealous, and even malignant animal. But it wasn't just me performing such pioneering procedures. The things I did could always be performed by my trainees and partners as well. I wasn't claiming to be a miracle worker or the only one who could get these remarkable results. It was not me having unusual talent; it was the techniques and the *system* we were able to develop, and the commitment to follow this system.

Even today, I often wonder why people were so skeptical of our work. Hard to know. It was partly professional jealousy. Some surgeons tried to replicate our work and were unsuccessful, possibly because they did not reproduce the many small details of our system. Occasionally, and in public, I would undiplomatically state that their lack of success was because they didn't perform the operations correctly. Of course, that bluntness did not win me many friends. Though I was sometimes shy, more often than not I was outspoken in the later phases of our limb salvage work. I knew then we were right, and I was troubled not to be believed.

Resentment of one's success by others is common. Human nature at work. Sometimes the resentment is subtle, but it is definitely there. For example, when I would get a major NIH grant, this good news was not always met with institutional support or acclaim. Clearly an accomplishment like that is good for the institution and all connected to it. It should be celebrated with a major press release, media interviews, and collegial congratulations. Unfortunately, we at Montefiore had an unusually egocentric hospital president who did not like disagreement from his subordinates and was particularly troubled when their differing advice proved to be correct. In my view, he didn't realize that his subordinates' success reflected well on him. He wanted all the glory.

For example, when we did the first US endovascular aortic aneurysm repair (EVAR) successfully, I went to him and said this game-changing achievement should get some publicity for Montefiore Medical Center—and that he could be the pitch man with the media. He did nothing, and the event went unnoticed in the New York City and national media when it should have been recognized as a great achievement for Montefiore.

The same held true for the Dean at Albert Einstein College of Medicine (AECOM), who seemed to resent and downplay any achievements of his vascular division at Montefiore. In fact, when we were awarded a large and very prestigious NIH Vascular Medicine Academic Award Grant, neither the President of Montefiore nor the Dean of AECOM acknowledged it publicly. All they did was fight over which institution should get the large amount of indirect funding.

To me, this was so short-sighted, small-minded, and sad. As I mentioned earlier, one reason medical administrators were skeptical of us was because of the additional medical costs accrued by our limb salvage techniques, particularly if the foot of the patient was extensively gangrenous. But our protocols worked. And the health and well-being of the patient was paramount to us. So we continued our limb salvage work even though it may not have been as profitable to our institution as other initiatives.

In 1981, after operating on 679 patients, we presented our findings to the ASA (American Surgical Association, the nation's oldest and most prestigious surgical organization), detailing our experience with limb salvage via bypasses or adjunctive surgical procedures, including PTA. Though most of our patients were quite sick, in most cases their salvaged limb functioned for as long as they lived.

All in all, after more than thirty-five years of practicing and promoting limb salvage surgery, I am very proud of our record. I and my colleagues in vascular surgery, interventional radiology, medicine, anesthesiology, and other specialties clearly led the way forward in establishing an entirely new field within the treatment of vascular diseases: namely, the aggressive saving of lower limbs facing a major amputation because of arteriosclerosis below the groin.

This field has now been joined by many other specialists in various disciplines: interventional cardiology, interventional radiology, angiology, and podiatry. All these specialists are now recognizing the importance of preventing major amputation in those patients with arteriosclerosis, diabetes, and end-stage renal disease. In fact, lower limb amputation due to these disease entities has recently been recognized as a worldwide health problem that needs to be addressed in a multispecialty manner to improve the lives of patients everywhere.

In the history of limb salvage, much has been accomplished, though it was disarming along the way to see how many hospital administrators and fellow surgeons maligned and doubted our aggressive surgical and endovascular procedures.

But no longer are we a voice in the wilderness, shunned by almost all except the patients whose limbs we saved. Finally, after more than forty years, vascular surgeons, cardiologists, and radiologists in the US and around the world have accepted our limb salvage techniques as both curative and cost effective for our health care systems. It is a song we sang decades ago. And now everyone is singing it.

In addition, our industry partners have helped substantially in our efforts to save limbs by providing ingenious new devices to reopen occluded arteries, greatly improving the applicability and effectiveness of endovascular treatments, thereby benefiting vast numbers of patients everywhere. Indeed, at present a majority of patients with threatened lower limbs can be treated endovascularly, although there will always be a need in some patients for the open bypass procedures we pioneered. The bottom line is that most lower limbs threatened with a major amputation because of poor arterial circulation can be saved by skilled and committed surgeons and physicians.

CHAPTER FIVE

THE ENDOVASCULAR REVOLUTION[9]

W ithin our bodies, we have an immensely complicated network of arteries, capillaries, and veins that comprise our circulatory system, with the heart as the pump that drives the blood through all of it.

If you were to lay out all of the arteries, capillaries and veins in one adult, end-to-end, they would stretch sixty thousand miles! And the capillaries, which are the smallest of the blood vessels, would make up about 80 percent of this length.

Miraculously, this closed system (meaning that the blood never leaves the network of arteries, veins, and capillaries) permits blood to circulate and transport nutrients, oxygen, carbon dioxide, hormones, and white blood cells to and from the cells in our bodies in order to provide nourishment and help fight diseases.

This complex vascular system is like a highway. It has to be wide open, allowing traffic (our blood) to flow. When there are no obstructions in the road, all is well. But when serious problems

---

9   The end of this chapter contains remarks relating to prevention and conservative treatment in vascular disease and the future of vascular surgery.

arise, like blockages or leaks in big arteries (or to a lesser extent veins), that's where a vascular surgeon may be needed.

Arterial obstructions or freed particles from a plaque can lead to a stroke or heart attack and death. Aneurysms or widened, weakened arteries can rupture and bleed internally. Blood vessels can be injured by bullets, knives, or blunt trauma. All these conditions can be treated or even averted with proper treatment from a vascular surgeon or vascular specialist.

Vascular surgeons have traditionally done their work to repair or overcome these conditions by performing open surgical operations, approaching blood vessels from their exterior via incisions in the abdomen, chest, neck, or extremities. These open surgical procedures include peripheral artery and aorta to distal artery bypasses around obstructions, aneurysm repairs or exclusions, and endarterectomies (a procedure to remove inner layers and plaque from a diseased artery that is obstructed or from which particles are breaking off and blocking smaller distal arteries). Endarterectomies are most often performed on the carotid artery in the neck to prevent plaque particles from going to the brain and causing a stroke

More recently, beginning in the 1960s, surgeons, radiologists, and cardiologists began to explore a new way of treating diseased arteries. This method involved approaching the damaged blood vessel from the *inside* of the vascular tree and fixing the diseased or damaged artery or vein from within. This new therapeutic approach was termed *endovascular surgery* or *endovascular treatment*.

It began in the 1960s when, as mentioned in the last chapter, a radiologist named Charles Dotter started to dilate obstructed leg arteries from within using tapered dilators introduced over a guidewire placed through the skin into the artery with just a hollow needle. Subsequently Andreas Gruentzig introduced balloon-tipped catheters to widen narrowed arteries in the heart and elsewhere. These procedures were termed *percutaneous transluminal angioplasties* (PTAs). Soon expandable metal cages or cylindrical frameworks, termed *stents*, were introduced percutaneously to keep the dilated or widened arteries open.

As also mentioned in the last chapter, I had become an enthusiast of endovascular treatments since I had heard Dotter at the New York Society for Cardiovascular Surgery when I was its president in 1979. As a result our interventional radiologist, Seymour Sprayregen, who I had prompted to visit with Dotter, began doing angioplasties and stents on our very sick limb salvage patients with multilevel disease.

In addition, because of my close association and friendship with Dr. Barry Katzen, a leading and pioneering interventional radiologist, I was invited to all his annual meetings in Miami, where I learned more about endovascular treatments and became even more enthusiastic about them—unlike most other vascular surgeons at the time.

At one of Dr. Katzen's meetings, in 1987, I heard Dr. Julio Palmaz present the theoretical ideas of a hugely talented and innovative Argentinian vascular surgeon, Dr. Juan Parodi, about treating aneurysms (widened weakened arteries). Parodi had proposed combining a stent and a prosthetic graft (introduced within the lumen of a more peripheral artery) to exclude an abdominal aortic aneurysm. His technique was much less invasive (and less risky) than the standard open operation of the day.

Although I found the concept fascinating, I elected not to pursue it at that point because I still thought interventional catheter-based endovascular procedures should only be done by interventional radiologists or by interventional cardiologists with the necessary catheter and guidewire skills. I also believed that only a small percentage of vascular patients would be best treated endovascularly. Little did I realize how dramatically my ideas would change five years later.

In the late 1980s, endovascular therapies were only feasible in a small proportion of patients, so they were no threat to vascular surgeons doing open surgery.

However, as you'll read in the pages ahead, this all changed in the early 1990s, when I persuaded Parodi to visit my group in New York City to help us perform the first endovascular aortic aneurysm repair (or EVAR) in North America using an endovascular stent-graft (EVG). My partnership with Parodi would gradually lead to a complete paradigm shift in the treatment of vascular diseases.

I viewed this development as a major turning point in US medical history, truly the beginning of the ENDOVASCULAR REVOLUTION. Why? Because I realized that the vast majority of vascular lesions could potentially be treated by endovascular procedures. That is why this chapter is a central one in the history of my professional life, as my role as a surgeon was completely transformed by my EVG experience. It led in a few years to an expansion from my role at Montefiore to a leadership position that would change the very nature of vascular surgery and vascular treatment.

As I begin this chapter about techniques and our pioneering advances in endovascular surgery, I will confess, strange as it sounds, that I was minimally trained as a vascular surgeon during my Peter Bent Brigham surgical residency! I was largely self-trained in most open vascular surgical procedures.

Why? Because in the 1960s, vascular surgery was not a specialty or even a sub-specialty. Back in those days, to acquire the skills needed to perform vascular surgery, you had to catch the training where you could. Some surgical trainees worked under the famed Dr. Michael DeBakey and his Texas colleagues, who were among the earliest surgeons to perform major arterial operations. Others trained under pioneering giants in vascular surgery like Dr. Edwin Jack Wylie, who was at the forefront of vascular surgical innovation at the University of California in San Francisco. (He was among the first to believe that vascular surgery should be a separate specialty.)

As for me, I had been trained in vascular surgery as part of my general surgery education under Dr. Chilton Crane and Dr. Richard Warren, both of whom had a passionate interest in it. But it was *still* only a part of general surgery. (Sadly, even today, vascular surgery is still a sub-specialty of general surgery, though it deserves to be a defined separate specialty—a topic to be covered later.)

When I came onto the scene at Montefiore in 1967, arterial procedures were still in their adolescence, with many of the modern-day technologies we take for granted today only on the horizon. In fact, up until 1992, all endovascular procedures except for arteriography were performed by the interventional radiologists at our institution with my full concurrence and support, as chief of vascular surgery. At that time, I was skilled in all open vascular surgical operations and had pioneered or improved many of them.

However, after our first EVAR case in 1992 with Juan Parodi and Claudio Schonholz (a story I will recount in a moment), everything in my mind and on my service changed dramatically. Most importantly, we started our own Montefiore surgeon-made endovascular stent-graft (EVG) program to handle mostly untreatable patients with aneurysms, occlusive and traumatic arterial lesions.

In the beginning, from 1993 to 1996, it was a bit like the wild west for us. For starters, we did everything ourselves, including making the EVGs, managing in our standard operating room our own ancient portable cine fluoroscope (which had been thrown out of the cardiology animal lab until we rescued it from the garbage). Also, our institution and the department of surgery would not let us purchase the approved balloon-expandable stents that were required to make the EVGs. Sometimes we had to obtain (procure) the stents from radiology by picking the locks to their storeroom!

Later, when commercial EVGs became available to treat some simple AAAs and we chose to use them, we had to pay for them ourselves because our institution (and our general surgery chairman) would not approve institutional payment for them.

Our early primitive surgeon-made EVGs were used to treat limb or life-threatening arterial problems in patients who otherwise would be difficult or impossible to treat. We made these EVGs by sewing balloon-expandable slotted metal cages or stents (Palmaz stents) to vascular grafts or tubes of expanded polytetrafluorethylene (PTFE or Teflon). The resulting EVG was then mounted on a balloon catheter (with the stent crimped on the balloon), and compressed so it would fit into a hollow plastic tube or introducer sheath small enough to pass through a peripheral artery to gain access to the problem or lesion being treated, often in a larger more central artery. This introducer sheath with the EVG and balloon catheter inside it was then passed over a previously placed guidewire and guided fluoroscopically into position to treat the arterial problem or lesion.

Once in position, the sheath was retracted and the balloon inflated to deploy the EVG and fix the lesion. Then the trick was to get the deflated balloon out without dislodging the EVG. Doing so was tricky but usually successful. The procedures were minimally invasive and remarkably effective.

Our introducer sheaths had tapered nose cones to protect the inside of arteries through which the devices were being inserted. Also, in our early work, the sheaths bled a lot because they had poor hemostatic mechanisms to block what was essentially an open tube in the lumen of a big artery. Early hemostatic mechanisms were minimally effective, whereas now much more effective hemostatic valves have been perfected by industry, and blood loss is much less.

Let's back up for a moment: You might ask, what attracted me to vascular surgery in the first place? From the start, I was always results-driven as a physician and surgeon, and could see that vascular surgical procedures could produce a big difference for severely ill patients.

From the beginning this was also dramatically true for EVGs. Actually, our results from the outset with primitive surgeon-made EVGs were remarkably effective in treating very difficult or otherwise untreatable patients! This was true with very challenging abdominal aortic aneurysms (AAAs) in patients too sick to tolerate any open operation. It was also true in our occlusive and traumatic cases.

In the beginning, we were just on the cusp of the golden age of EVAR with EVGs first fabricated for a tiny number of patients by us and a few other surgeons, and shortly thereafter by industry. However, EVAR would one day surpass open aortic surgery as the most common technique for repair of AAAs. In fact, by 2010, EVAR, a procedure designed to exclude the AAA from the circulation by lining it with an EVG accounted for 78 percent of all elective US AAA repairs. The benefits of EVAR over open repair were many.

The procedure was minimally invasive, requiring less anesthesia and only a small groin incision. It therefore caused less pain, less overall trauma, less dissection, less damage to adjacent organs, less bleeding, less hypothermia, less large vessel injury, and overall less patient risk than open surgical repairs done through a long abdominal incision. The end result was that there was less stress on the patient and less time spent in the ICU and in post-operative hospital care.

But nobody knew *any* of this would be true at the time we were starting out with EVGs at Montefiore in the early '90s, confident in our belief that patients who were morbidly ill or had no other therapeutic option could be made better by a less invasive procedure.

Then there was the treatment of ruptured AAAs, an area in which we were clearly *the* pioneer, as we performed at Montefiore the first EVAR for a ruptured AAA in the world.

Prior to EVAR, vascular surgeons (including me) had at best a 40 to 50 percent early mortality rate treating ruptured AAAs with open surgery. But with EVAR the thirty-day mortality rate was reduced to around 20 percent. Importantly, some ruptured AAA patients who could not be treated by any open operation were left untreated and would always die. Yet such patients could still be treated by EVAR and often survive.

Furthermore, even with elective open repair of AAAs, the thirty-day mortality was about 3–5 percent. But as we would discover, with EVAR the early mortality rate was about 1.6 percent. These early mortality benefits for EVAR were astounding.

Also, along with our early work with EVAR beginning in 1992, my colleagues and I were pioneers in performing the first endovascular graft (EVG) repairs of a variety of other arterial lesions—aneurysms, occlusions, and traumatic injuries (knife and gunshot wounds) of arteries other than the aorta. We successfully performed many of these EVG cases—often in emergent situations—because we were able to quickly fabricate our own surgeon-made EVGs.

In addition to performing the first elective EVAR in the US and North America and because we could then make our own EVGs, we were able to perform the first EVG treatments for occlusive disease, iliac and popliteal artery aneurysms, EVAR for ruptured AAAs, subclavian artery injuries and aneurysms, and many other vascular lesions.

Abdominal aortic aneurysms (AAAs) have always been a particularly interesting and sometimes challenging entity for vascular surgeons to treat. An aneurysm is an abnormal, progressive dilatation of an artery, vein, or the aorta. The condition is most common in the abdominal aorta, and when large, it carries a substantial risk for rupture with massive bleeding and certain death without treatment. Open operations could save about half of such patients reaching a hospital, but mortality for open repair with aortic rupture remained high despite all efforts to lower it.

This irreducible high mortality for open repair of ruptured AAAs always motivated me to find a better way to treat this common and challenging condition. So, when a less invasive way to treat it appeared possible with EVGs, it was only natural that we wanted to try it. Moreover, our surgeon-made EVG, which was a one-size-fits-most, could be sterilized and kept on our operating room shelf to treat an emergent condition like a ruptured AAA. This was a huge asset in the early days of EVAR since the available industry-made grafts, which were size and length dependent, had to be ordered and sent to the institution. This required an unacceptable delay of many hours or days. Because of the immediate availability of our EVG, it was not surprising that we were able to perform the first EVAR in the world for a ruptured AAA on April 21, 1994.

In the early days of our EVG program at Montefiore, we only did EVAR on patients who could not have an open repair, which limited the number of cases we did. We also performed only a few AAA cases early on because we did not have easy access to larger Palmaz stents. But smaller FDA-approved balloon-expandable (Palmaz) stents were available. It was these that we used to make EVGs suitable for treating lesions in smaller arteries—aneurysmal, occlusive, and traumatic.

Because of their experimental nature, we largely used these surgeon-made EVGs to treat patients who could not be treated by a standard open or endovascular procedure and who had an urgent life- or limb-threatening arterial lesion. Later on, industry-made EVGs became available for treating AAAs and we used them—often in clinical trials. The AAA patients that could be treated by industry-made grafts were usually easier and with less challenging anatomy. So even until the late 90s, we still had to make our own grafts for the more difficult or emergency AAAs or other lesion cases. Then as time passed industry-made EVGs became more widely available for AAAs and other lesions. These industry-made EVGs were generally better and could also be stocked in operating rooms for urgent cases. Thus, surgeon-made EVGs are now rarely needed and used.

In 1992, my surgical team at Montefiore included a promising young vascular surgeon named Dr. Michael L. Marin, who was just two months out of fellowship training with us. Dr. Marin played a major role in our endovascular graft program, and made many important contributions to it. Today I am proud that he is the chairman of the entire department of surgery at Mount Sinai Hospital, one of New York's most outstanding medical centers.

In August of that year, Marin and I were called on to treat a seventy-six-year-old man, diagnosed with a large (7.5 centimeters, or 3 inches, in diameter) painful AAA. In addition, he suffered oxygen-dependent pulmonary insufficiency and severe inoperable coronary artery disease with recurrent ventricular arrhythmias.

Despite all these issues, the patient was mentally alert, optimistic, and wanted his threatening AAA fixed. Yet all those who evaluated him deemed him a prohibitively high risk for an open AAA repair.

But because the patient appeared to have favorable anatomy for an EVAR procedure, with a long neck of normal aorta proximal to his AAA and below the arteries to his kidneys, a well-defined distal neck, and large straight iliac arteries, we immediately thought of doing a less invasive endovascular repair. However, we did not know how to do it!

Up until this point, only five EVAR procedures had ever been performed—all in Argentina by Juan C. Parodi. Yes, I had studied articles describing endovascular repair in animals and was fascinated by them, but that's as far as my expertise went.

When Marin and I spoke about our patient's inoperability and our technical inability to perform an EVAR, we both said, "Let's go to Argentina!"

Why? Because we knew of the pioneering work of Dr. Parodi, an Argentinian vascular surgeon (trained at the Cleveland Clinic) who had published a single article on his first cases of EVAR, although few paid much heed to his work at the time.

We knew that in 1990 Parodi had performed the first successful EVG repair of an abdominal aortic aneurysm on a friend of Carlos Menem, then president of Argentina. It was a procedure that involved the placement of a tubular EVG into the AAA to exclude it from the high-pressure arterial circulation. In contrast to open surgical repair, Parodi's EVARs only required a small groin incision, minimal anesthesia, and no dissection within the abdomen. Recovery was rapid and relatively painless.

When I called Dr. Parodi, he picked up right away because he was aware of our vascular surgery symposium and wanted to come to it, as his innovations were generally disregarded by other vascular surgeons. I asked him if we could travel to Buenos Aires to learn how to do the EVAR procedure. He said he had no more such procedures scheduled.

"Then why don't you come to New York and help us do the case?" I asked him. He answered that he would review our patient's x-rays (angiograms and CT scans) and be in touch.

Beyond Parodi's initial hesitation about coming to Montefiore, there was some resistance from within our institution as well, the usual pushback to "change." But because I was the chief of vascular surgery and the chairman of surgery at the time, I had the leverage to allow Parodi and his interventional radiologist colleague, Claudio Schonholz to participate in our case.

There were many mishaps all along the way. For example, when we sent Parodi the x-rays, they were somehow lost. We then sent another set. Mission accomplished. After reviewing them, Parodi told us that he was coming to a meeting in Milwaukee, and that we could come and discuss the case with him. I had an emergency in New York and could not make the trip. So Marin went, presented our case with his suitable anatomy, and convinced Parodi to perform the first EVAR outside of Argentina with us. At this point, we also invited Dr. Parodi to give a talk at our annual vascular surgery symposium. It was agreed that he would speak at the meeting and then come to Montefiore a few days later to help us perform the EVAR on our patient.

To provide the funding for the Argentineans' trip to New York City, I fortunately had the resources we needed from an unrestricted grant from the Manning Foundation. Drs. Parodi and Schonholz were accompanied by their device engineer, Hector Barone (who would construct the EVG and deployment system). Although it was a very expensive trip, it was certainly worth it to us and the patient.

After much back-and-forth negotiation about hotel and flight arrangements, Parodi and his colleagues flew to New York in November 1992. Two days after speaking at our meeting, his team arrived at our hospital, as promised, to lead the operation on our ailing patient.

Although our plan for doing the procedure was in place, many logistic issues had to be resolved before we could do the case. One was getting permission from Johnson & Johnson Interventional Systems (JJIS) to use a large balloon-expandable (Palmaz-like) stent since JJIS had the rights to both Palmaz's and Parodi's patents. The company was concerned that our use of a large Palmaz-like stent without an Investigational Device Exemption from the Food and Drug Administration (FDA) would impair the company's ability to get FDA approval to implant smaller Palmaz-Schatz balloon-expandable stents in the coronary arteries of the heart.

So Marin and I met the JJIS president, Marvin Woodall, and their director of new products, Paul Marshall—also a friend of mine—in the Newark airport Marriott restaurant. They kept saying no to our request to be allowed to use a Palmaz-like stent. We had them pinned in a corner table and wouldn't let them out as the evening dragged on. After four hours, the other customers had left. The waiters had all the chairs up on the tables and were closing. Finally, Woodall said, "I am exhausted. Do whatever the hell you want." So we went ahead.

Yet, upon Parodi's arrival at Montefiore on November 22 of that year, it didn't look like it was going to happen after all. Parodi and Schonholz took one look at the primitive fluoroscopy equipment in our operating room and said "NO!" Our equipment was not adequate. No way would they participate in the case. However, with the life of our patient in the balance, we made the equipment work adequately and talked Parodi and Schonholz into letting us go forward with the procedure.

It was amazing watching them in action: A 22-mm in diameter knitted Dacron graft was sewn to a large balloon-expandable (Palmaz-like) stent. The resulting stent and EVG were mounted on a balloon catheter and compressed to fit within a large plastic sheath so it would fit within the lumen of the femoral artery in the patient's groin. The resulting device was then passed over a guidewire into position fluoroscopically so that the graft-covered distal half of the single proximal stent was entirely within the 2.5-cm-long non-aneurysmal neck of the AAA. The sheath was then retracted and the stent deployed by inflation of the balloon on which it was mounted. No distal stent was employed. Despite that, aneurysm exclusion was demonstrated by intraoperative angiography and ultrasound sonography. The prominent AAA pulse was markedly reduced, and the patient's pain was totally relieved.

On that fall day in 1992, the operation succeeded brilliantly and we had made history at Montefiore, performing the first EVAR outside of Argentina.

And would you believe that the next day our elderly patient was up in a chair reading *Playboy* magazine! (We have the photo to prove it.) Despite all his serious comorbidities, our lively patient went on to survive comfortably without AAA symptoms for many months before succumbing to his heart disease and its rhythm problems.

The success of that procedure was truly the beginning of the endovascular revolution in the treatment of vascular lesions. It was both a game-changing landmark event for me, for Marin, and for Montefiore as well, making us the first US hospital to perform a less invasive AAA repair with an EVG.

Our Montefiore vascular surgeons, in collaboration with our interventional radiologists and Argentinian colleagues, thereafter embarked on a program of endovascular grafting for the treatment of aneurysms at various locations, traumatic arterial lesions, and aorto-iliac and femoral occlusive disease.

Indeed, when I saw what we were able to do for our AAA patient in an otherwise hopeless circumstance, I had an epiphany. I thought, "My God, this is going to change our vascular world. If an endovascular graft worked this well in a very sick patient with a symptomatic and threatening AAA, imagine the benefit for a wide range of patients." In subsequent years, that epiphany fortunately spread to the rest of vascular surgery and other vascular specialties, albeit more slowly than I would have liked.

Yes, I had always been enthusiastic about balloon angioplasties, stents, and other endovascular techniques performed by our radiologists. However, this case and our subsequent success with surgeon-made EVGs for a variety of arterial lesions, that would ordinarily require a big and morbid open operation, made me realize that the availability of EVGs and other endovascular technologies would likely lead to a paradigm shift in the treatment of vascular pathology—the endovascular revolution that I referred to earlier.

"In fact," I thought to myself, "vascular surgeons better stop referring their endovascular procedures to interventional radiologists and learn how to do them." Otherwise we would all be out of a job and our specialty of vascular surgery would become extinct.

What does this mean? I worried that we as vascular surgeons would never survive as a specialty or "species," and that we would be replaced by interventional specialists (interventional radiologists and interventional cardiologists) unless we mastered endovascular techniques to treat our patients. Indeed, we *would* have become greatly diminished or extinct if it weren't for me and a handful of other vascular surgeons who realized the potential of endovascular treatments. More on this in a moment.

Getting back to 1992: In the aftermath of Dr. Parodi's first visit to Montefiore and the astounding turnaround of our patient, we brought Parodi and his partners back from Argentina to Montefiore a few months later to help us perform three additional EVAR cases (all on very sick inoperable patients). Only two of these three patients survived, with only one doing really well for a long time.

Thereafter Parodi advised us (me and Marin) on how he made the grafts and deployment systems. We then modified what we had learned about these devices and started making them ourselves. Most of our early EVGs were made with approved stents and vascular grafts. However, for a long time we did not have FDA approval for combining these approved devices, which were clearly experimental and totally beyond the standard of care.

I realized at the time that I was taking responsibility for doing this, and that I was exposing myself to substantial medico-legal and

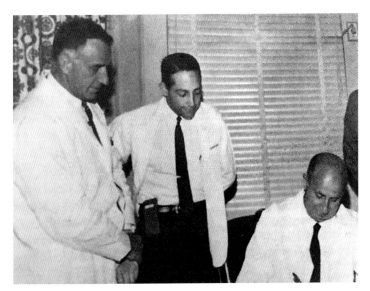

Dr. Veith, as chief resident at Peter Bent Brigham Hospital in 1962, with Dr. Francis D. Moore, left, and Dr. Robert Zollinger Sr., right, both preeminent surgical leaders of the time.

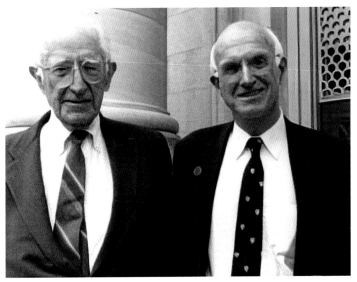

Dr. Moore, left, with Joseph Murray, a future Nobel laureate.

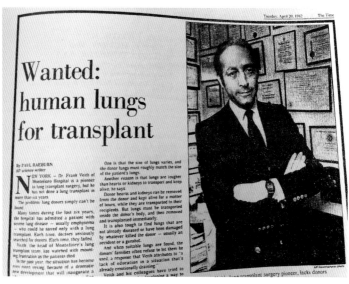

A 1982 feature article documenting the difficulties in obtaining donor lungs for transplantation, as featured in the *New York Times*. (Associated Press)

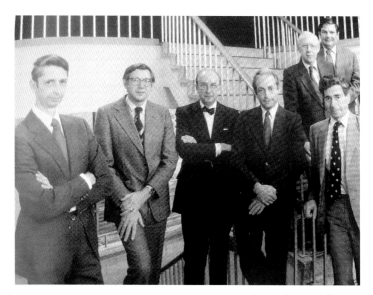

Pioneers in clinical organ transplantation. Front row from left: Randall Griepp (heart transplantation); Frank Stuart (kidney and liver transplantation). Front row from right: Sir Roy Calne (kidney transplantation and immunosuppression); Frank Veith (lung transplantation). Back row from right: Anthony Monaco (kidney transplantation); Marvin Gliedman (pancreas transplantation).

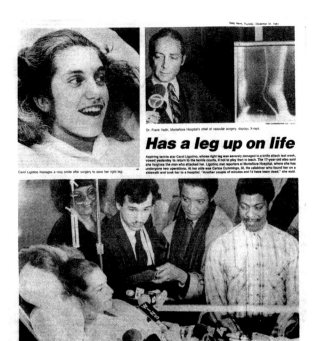

Carol Ligotino, tennis star, after the arterial bypass which saved her right leg from amputation after a knife attack left her with a limb-threatening wound. (*New York Daily News*, 1981)

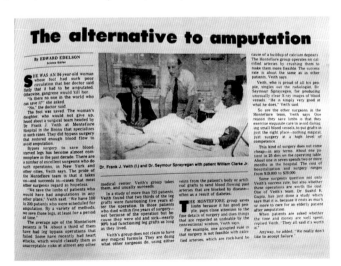

Article on a limb-saving angioplasty and bypass. (*New York Daily News*, 1983)

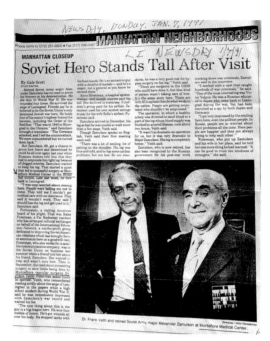

Article on a Soviet World War II hero who came to the US to have his lower limb saved by a difficult bypass operation. (*Newsday*, 1991)

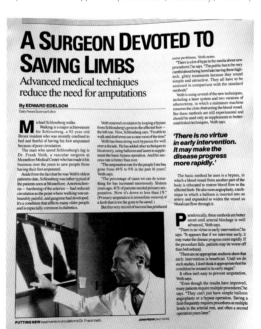

Article on new techniques to avoid lower limb amputations. (*New York Daily News*, 1990)

A Life-Saving Lung

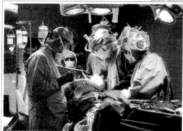

Scott Wilson of Boca Raton, Fla., was "as close to being dead as he could be without being dead," according to Surgeon Frank Veith of Montefiore Medical Center in New York City. Wilson, 25, a landscaper and father of four, was spraying weeds with the herbicide paraquat on Aug. 30, when the equipment apparently malfunctioned and he accidentally inhaled the toxic chemical. Paraquat lodges in the muscle tissue and travels in the blood to the lungs, where it does continual damage as long as it remains in the body. After steadily declining in a Florida hospital, Wilson was transferred to Montefiore in a final effort to save his life. There, doctors continued to remove the poison from his system by filtering his blood through charcoal. But it was too late: the paraquat had already done drastic harm to Wilson's lungs. His only hope: a lung transplant.

Since 1963, doctors around the world have attempted 50 such operations (seven of which were performed by Veith at Montefiore), but only in the past few years, with the introduction of cyclosporine, a drug that helps prevent the rejection of foreign tissue, have patients survived more than a year. At present the only survivor besides Wilson is another paraquat victim, who had two lungs transplanted in separate operations several weeks ago in Toronto. One limiting factor for lung transplants is the lack of suitable donors. Wilson, however, was lucky. The lungs of Thomas Riso, 19, an auto-accident victim who matched Wilson in size and blood type, became available. Riso's right lung was infected with pneumonia, but the left was healthy enough to be transferred. It was artificially inflated, drained of blood and filled instead with a cold fluid that kept it at a temperature close to freezing during the 93-min. interval between excision and implantation. The entire procedure took six hours and involved five surgeons, three anesthesiologists, two pulmonary specialists and 15 nurses and technicians. At week's end Wilson, though still in critical condition, was awake, responsive and watching television.

Wilson's new lung lies on his chest before Veith, center, implants it

76

Time magazine article on a transplant to try to save a young man dying of paraquat damage to his lungs, October 1982.

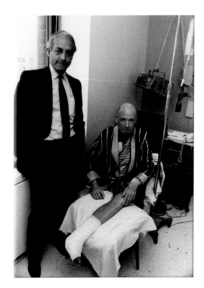

Dr. Veith with a limb salvage patient after a successful bypass operation, 1982.

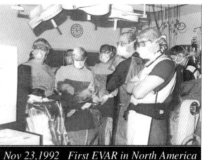

Nov 23,1992   First EVAR in North America
Montefiore Hospital, Bronx, New York

Operating room photo from the first US endovascular aortic aneurysm repair, November 22, 1992.

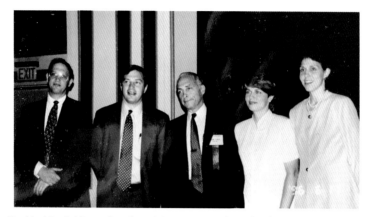

Dr. Veith's children after the 1996 SVS Presidential Address.
From left: Richard, Frank. From right: Katherine and Margaret.

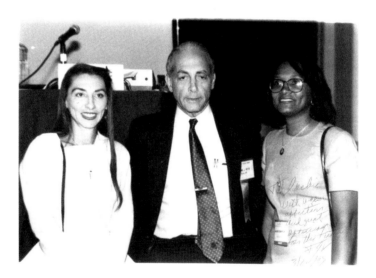

Valued colleagues: on the left, Julie Harris, and on the right, Jackie Simpson,
after the 1996 SVS Presidential Address.

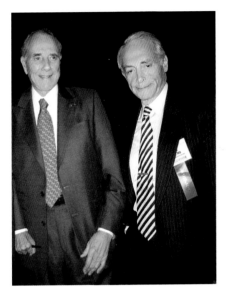

With senator and presidential candidate Bob Dole after his address to the VEITHsymposium, November 2003.

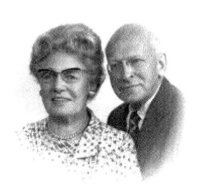

Dr. Veith's mother, Joan, and father, Frank, 1960.

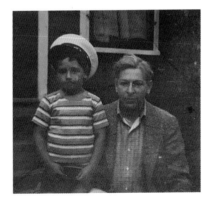

Dr. Veith at age four with uncle James.

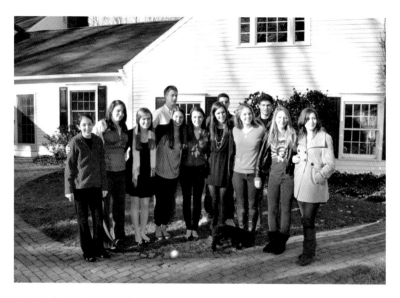

Dr. Veith's twelve grandchildren, November 2012.

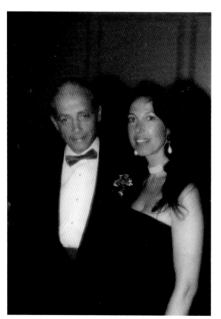

Carol and Frank Veith after the
1996 SVS Presidential Address.

regulatory (FDA) risks. However, I felt that these risks were worth taking because of the good results we were obtaining and because of the importance of this work in improving patient care. I also felt that these early EVG experiences would be the spark that ignited an endovascular revolution, which would lead to a paradigm shift for the better in the way vascular lesions were going to be treated around the world.

After our first cases with Parodi, our EVG program moved swiftly forward. Mike Marin and I made our own EVGs and delivery systems to treat an increasing number of AAAs as well as a variety of other arterial lesions in various parts of the body. Almost all were used in difficult circumstances on patients in whom no other open surgical or endovascular treatment was possible.

With AAAs, the AAA was excluded from the circulation; for occlusions, the lumen was restored; and for lacerated or destroyed arteries (knife or gun wounds), the defect in the artery was lined by the prosthetic PTFE graft so the bleeding stopped. Our early experiences definitely were game-changers in vascular surgery.

I remember one vivid example of how using our new techniques saved a life. In 1994, I got an emergency phone call from our affiliated city institution, Jacobi Hospital. They had just admitted a drug dealer who had been shot multiple times in the right shoulder and chest. He was in shock, actively bleeding from the gunshot wound of his right subclavian artery.

I immediately told the emergency doc at Jacobi to get the patient to the operating room and set up the fluoroscope. I then rushed to our radiology department and grabbed an assortment of Palmaz stents and a variety of balloon catheters, guidewires, etc. I put these in a shopping bag! (I already had PTFE [Teflon] grafts from our operating room.)

I then raced to the front of Montefiore Medical Center where

I got a gypsy cab because no regular yellow taxis would come into the Bronx in 1994. In ten minutes, I was in the Jacobi operating room with the patient who, by then, had a very low blood pressure of 50 mm Hg.

With the help of the interventional radiologist, we got access through a femoral artery in the groin and passed a catheter over a guidewire into the right subclavian artery in the patient's shoulder to obtain an arteriogram. The test revealed an injury to the subclavian artery with major bleeding.

We then placed an over-the-wire balloon catheter in the subclavian artery proximal to the injury and inflated the balloon. This stopped the bleeding. I then took a small Palmaz stent, sewed a segment of PTFE graft to it. (This was the hardest part of the procedure because the interstices of the stent were very small and hard to see, especially with many observers in the operating room watching closely.)

I compressed the stent and graft onto a balloon and put it in a sheath (tube) with a tapered tip glued to the balloon tip by crazy glue. Next, I got open access to the brachial artery, passed a wire proximally with it easily traversing the damaged subclavian artery injury. Over this wire I then passed the sheath containing the balloon mounted EVG that I had made.

By retracting the sheath, the EVG was exposed. I shot an angiogram through the sheath to show that the stent-graft was in position to cover the defect in the subclavian artery. Then I inflated the balloon to deploy the stent-graft. An angiogram showed that the arterial defect was covered. We deflated the balloon in the proximal subclavian artery, did another arteriogram to show there was no further bleeding, removed the sheath, wire and catheters, repaired the small defect in the brachial artery, and closed the one-inch incision at the elbow.

This was all much quicker and safer than the complex open surgical procedure required to get exposure of the subclavian artery. Moreover, I followed the patient for many years, and the EVG remained patent with no complications. However, when I presented this case and other examples of EVGs to repair axillary/subclavian artery injuries at an American College of Surgeons meeting, I was greeted with disdain and almost ridicule for spoiling a good open operative repair.

But nothing stopped us. During the early '90s, we treated more than 150 such cases, all with different arterial pathology in patients who could not otherwise be treated by traditional open operations or endovascular procedures (stents and balloon catheters). Such patients included those with high-risk symptomatic or threatening AAAs, ruptured AAAs, aneurysms in other locations difficult to reach by open exposures, very difficult limb salvage patients otherwise facing an imminent amputation (usually after multiple previous procedural failures), and difficult traumatic arterial injuries like subclavian disruptions and arteriovenous fistulas. Even in these challenging circumstances, these primitive surgeon-made EVGs proved to be surprisingly successful.

Much to our surprise and delight, despite the primitive surgeon-made technology, most of the procedures worked. The patients not only survived, but thrived. Still, rarely we also had several jolting and even disastrous complications as we were discovering pitfalls that had never been described or noted before. One such case involved a taut guidewire injury to a subclavian artery during a very difficult EVAR procedure. We could not see the guidewire fluoroscopically because the wire had come apart due to the tension on it. Today, with improved technology and skills, these bad outcomes rarely happen anymore.

Clearly all these points were true with EVAR, which was better, safer, and simpler in some patients—both with elective and ruptured AAAs. This had been my opinion from the outset. However, others in the field disagreed about the superior nature of EVAR and the use of EVGs in other circumstances. These opinions were sometimes supported by randomized controlled trials (RCTs) that had major flaws and biases. This was a situation we addressed in an article that examined three randomized controlled trials concluding that thirty-day mortality outcomes after EVAR for ruptured AAAs are no better than those after open repair. However, as we wrote in the article, "we are concerned that in all three trials these conclusions are rendered unjustified or misleading because of serious flaws or misinterpretation of the trial data."[10]

The major flaw in one of the RCTs was that less than half the patients in the endovascular strategy group were treated with EVAR, with more than half being treated with open repair. Or as we stated in the article: "Of the 316 patients initially randomized to the Endovascular Strategy group, only 154 (less than half) were actually treated by EVAR . . ." The rest had an open repair or no treatment.

In short, I believe that comparing the results or outcomes in the two groups open vs. endo) was not justified. It seems doctors should know better than slanting their conclusions in this way. However, all of us are subject to biases. And I believe some of these misleading

---

10   Veith FJ, Rockman CB, "The recent randomized trials of EVAR versus open repair for ruptured abdominal aortic aneurysms are misleading," *Vascular* 2015; 23(2): 217–219.

conclusions go back to the anti-endovascular bias which many older vascular surgeons have had. This was common in the earlier days, and sadly it occasionally still exists, albeit rarely.

Despite resistance and imperfect scientific data, the endovascular revolution was now fully underway, transforming the way vascular lesions were treated all over the industrialized world, though open surgery was still the best alternative for some patients, and for a few it is the only alternative.

As we began to perform successfully more endovascular EVG procedures for AAAs and other vascular lesions, we recorded the results of each case in great detail. Despite my usual caution about overstating good results and my uncertainty about the long-term value of EVGs, our initial short-term results were so promising that I thought we should present our work at conferences and publish our results widely in multiple medical journals.

My goal was to inspire other vascular surgeons to share our enthusiasm for this new way of treating arterial lesions. Moreover, many of our early cases justified publication because they were the first of their kind to be performed.

On the subject of publication, I usually let my junior associates take the lead as first author of these papers because I wanted to promote their careers, a subject we will cover in the mentorship chapter. In addition to everyone's hard work, this sharing attitude was an unusual hallmark of my career at Montefiore. It turned out to be a major reason our group was able to achieve as much as it did.

While some of my associates appreciated my attitude and generosity, some did not. A few were even so jealous of our progress that they tried to take me down. Once again, I encountered an unsavory or jungle-like aspect of human nature—the Brutus-Caesar syndrome. But we plowed ahead and appeared at many key national and international conferences, giving talks all over the world on what we were able to do and how we did it. Some believed us and our enthusiasm, many others did not.

Here is one example of such skepticism. Our group plus Parodi submitted an abstract for presentation in 1993 to the prestigious Society for Vascular Surgery (SVS). This abstract described the first thirty cases of successful EVGs in patients. Shockingly, the abstract didn't survive the first perfunctory cut by the SVS program committee. It was just dismissed as absurd wackiness. But then, also in 1993, we tried to present our work to a group of younger vascular surgery leaders in what was called the Vascular Surgery Biology Club. All the members were my good friends and rising stars in vascular surgery. However, we had trouble getting our work heard because there was only one presentation per year, and that spot had already been given to a basic science talk on co-culturing endothelial cells and smooth muscle cells. But I did not want to wait another year. I felt our data was so important and game changing that it should be shared as soon as possible. So I persuaded the club secretary to allow me ten minutes during the cocktail hour to present what were then our unexpectedly good results.

Surprisingly and disappointingly, no one in the audience found my presentation credible. I had brought Dr. Parodi and Dr. Marin to the meeting as my guests. But aside from them, nobody else believed what we were saying. Uniformly, these relatively young hot shots, supposed leaders in vascular surgery, were intensely skeptical of our good results in these seemingly impossible cases (which *had* been impossible to treat by any other means). They thought we were either lying, crazy, or wackos.

As one of them told me: "This is never going to work. And if it does work, you shouldn't be doing it." The implication of some was that these techniques would not work and even if they did, vascular surgeons should not be doing them. Instead, interventional radiologists or cardiologists should be performing these procedures.

And my comeback was: "Well, what if they *do* work?! If that is the case and we don't start learning how to do them now, we vascular surgeons will be out of business."

Most of my vascular surgery colleagues in other institutions insisted that standard open operations were the best way to treat vascular lesions, and there was no room for improvement. They simply couldn't believe there was another better and safer way to approach them, namely from within the lumen or inside channel of arteries and veins rather than by dissecting them out from their outside and fixing them.

To further illustrate the kind of resistance we encountered for our pioneering work, let's zero in on the year 1995: In the fall of that year, I was appointed head of a committee to provide endovascular training for vascular surgical trainees. Toward that effort, I gained the assistance of a few other iconoclastic vascular surgeons, all out of the mainstream of the specialty, who were *already* embracing endovascular techniques.

However, the president of the Association of Program Directors in Vascular Surgery (who was also a good friend) said such training was unnecessary because EVGs and EVAR wouldn't work. I was dismayed to say the least, more so when he summarily *fired* me as the committee chairman of endovascular training, saying I was too "enthusiastic."

I was angry and immediately challenged him: "What if these procedures *work*? Where will our trainees be in future years and what state will our specialty be in if we're not ready?" He said it wouldn't matter to him because he would be retired in five years!

That only illustrated the resistance we faced. As a result of his bias and resistance, endovascular training was not included in the vascular surgery training curriculum for several years.

One of the best summaries of our early work with EVGs was presented in 1994. At the time I was fortunate enough to be the president of the Eastern Vascular Society. For this important event, the topic of my presidential address was "Transluminally placed endovascular stented grafts (or TPEGs) and their impact on vascular surgery." (TPEGs was the descriptive term I used for EVGs at the time.)

In that presidential address (reprinted in the Appendix), I started by talking about how vascular surgery was being buffeted by the winds of change, and that our success rate with EVGs for treating vascular lesions was very positive. I reported that thirty-seven of the forty-three first patients who were treated with EVGs were doing well with patent functioning grafts ten months after their procedure. Only two patients died from complications of their procedure despite their severe comorbidities that rendered them unsuitable for any other treatment. Despite the preponderance of encouraging data, almost none of my colleagues and certainly not the older leaders agreed with what I was saying. They were doubtful that these newer less-invasive endovascular procedures could work as well or better than established open operations.

I posed this question in my address: "Why are we all so agitated by EVGs when we [vascular surgeons] were not as disturbed by balloon angioplasty or even the premature hype about endovascular lasers? Simply stated, balloon angioplasty was applicable to only a small percentage of our surgical cases, and lasers never worked very well. However, EVGs are a potentially better method to treat a major fraction of our surgical cases."

But the vascular surgery veterans there did not want to believe our results, because they would transform their specialty and their practices. They feared that physicians like us who could perform EVAR and EVGs would lead to them losing their patients. Money was also indirectly an issue because some established vascular surgeons didn't want to interrupt their income stream long enough to learn new skills.

I correctly predicted in that presidential address and accompanying article that "furious turf battles or war" were inevitable between vascular surgeons and interventional specialists (radiologists and cardiologists). These specialties would vie with vascular surgery to perform procedures involving a new technology like EVGs.

But as I wrote: "The crucial step in avoiding this conflict is for both groups to retreat from these extremist views, remove the fear factor, and reassure each other by word and deed that mutual destruction is not a goal. Interventional radiologists must be reassured that vascular surgeons do not intend to take over diagnostic angiography, balloon angioplasty, and stent placement as they currently exist. Vascular surgeons must be assured that they will be able to perform EVG insertions as they replace open vascular operative procedures." But many of our colleagues continued to believe that vascular surgeons shouldn't be performing these procedures! Instead, holding onto their territory, they insisted that interventional radiologists and interventional cardiologists were the ones who should be performing EVAR and other endovascular procedures.

To sum it up, despite what I had to say in 1994 at that Eastern Vascular Society meeting, few in our field listened. Indeed, my presentation was largely met with disbelief, skepticism, and disinterest. The old guard was resistant to that kind of innovation, greeting our and Parodi's game-changing advances with predictable negativity. They felt as if we were traipsing on a perfectly good vascular treatment system of the past and present. Some even told us that what we were doing was ethically "wrong."

For example, two years later when I was president of the SVS, the secretary of that society and a friend, Jonathan Towne, called me to say I shouldn't be performing EVG and EVAR procedures with surgeon-made stent-grafts because it put me in legal jeopardy and might embarrass the SVS. I acknowledged that he was partially right, that I was taking risks, but that I thought it was the right thing to do—that these risks were worth taking and could lead to improved care for patients and save lives and limbs.

Slowly, some enlightened (particularly younger) vascular surgeons were persuaded by our talks, publications, and results. And EVGs and EVAR gradually caught on a bit. However, the vast majority were not convinced by the mid- or late 1990s.

Still no matter what anyone said, I knew in my heart that EVGs and EVAR were going to be a game-changer and that vascular surgeons had to get involved to prevent interventional specialists from taking the lead in this technology. In other words, if vascular surgeons did not embrace endovascular skills and techniques, they would rapidly be replaced by interventionalists in cardiology and radiology, and vascular surgery would become diminished or extinct as a specialty. We would be out of the game. And I did not want this to happen.

I made this point most emphatically in 1996 as the president of the Society for Vascular Surgery. My presidential address (reprinted in the Appendix) to the esteemed SVS was titled: "Charles Darwin and Vascular Surgery." It was a speech that certainly went against the grain as it dealt with the evolution of vascular surgery and how we had to change and evolve as a specialty in order to survive and prosper.

For starters, you might wonder: What was the possible relevance Darwin, the famous English naturalist and the father of the theory of evolution, could have to vascular surgery?!

I first recounted Darwin's theory of evolution by natural selection, first formulated in his book, *On the Origin of Species by Means of Natural Selection, or the Preservation of Favoured Races in the Struggle for Life*. In this classic volume, published first in 1859, Darwin pointed out the process by which organisms change over time as a result of changes in heritable physical or behavioral traits. Changes that allow an organism to better adapt to its environment will help it survive and have more offspring.

Using Darwin's work as a metaphor, I likened specialties to species and indicated that medical specialties, like species, had to evolve and become different from their ancestors if they were to avoid extinction and survive. I also made three predictions and associated recommendations for future survival adaptations. Two of these recommendations proved to be unworkable or unsuccessful. One proved to be remarkably right.

One errant recommendation was that we work collaboratively and congenially with interventional radiologists or cardiologists in dedicated vascular centers. The idea was that we could learn from one another, sharing our skill sets for the betterment of all. That kumbaya recommendation proved unworkable because of medical tribalism, competitive human nature, and greed. The three specialties involved in treating blood vessels—vascular surgeons, interventional radiologists, and interventional cardiologists—all wanted to be dominant and in control of patients and the resultant dollars earned.

A second recommendation was that vascular surgery become more independent as a specialty, separate from general and cardiac surgery, just like the specialties of neurosurgery, orthopedics, urology, obstetrics and gynecology, plastic surgery, and cardiothoracic surgery.

As I wrote: "Vascular Surgery's evolution and separation are inevitable because its members are better adapted, more 'fit' by virtue of training and experience to care for vascular disease patients . . . Darwin would predict that forces of evolution will result in the distinct separation of our specialty . . . which would eliminate much conflict of interest and probably be best for all concerned," most notably the vascular patients that we served.

With that point in mind, I knew that we, as vascular surgeons, needed to separate administratively and gain an American Board of Medical Specialties (ABMS)–recognized governing board and Residency Review Committee (RRC). A vigorous attempt to accomplish this was made between 1996 and 2007, but failed, a topic to be covered in Chapter 6. As a result, vascular surgery still remains a subservient subspecialty in North America, although it is not in most other parts of the civilized world.

My third recommendation in 1996 was prophetic and fared better. I predicted an endovascular revolution and recommended that vascular surgeons *had* to become competent in all endovascular techniques, embracing and practicing these new techniques. Otherwise, they would risk extinction.

In this 1996 address, I predicted that within ten years, 40 percent to 70 percent of the open operations we were then doing would be replaced by endovascular procedures. And many of the remaining "open" operations would be improved and simplified by using the endovascular adjuncts that were available (such as catheters, guidewires, sheaths, digital fluoroscopy, balloons, stents, and EVGs). All this certainly turned out to be true in spades!

Accordingly, in this 1996 address I recommended that vascular surgeons, if they wished to survive, had to become endo-competent, acquiring catheter-guidewire-imaging skills that would enable them to perform all sorts of endovascular treatments.

Although this recommendation was greeted with disdain and strongly resisted by many senior vascular surgeons at the time, this resistance was gradually overcome. Our specialty has embraced the endovascular revolution and become endo-competent. This is why vascular surgery is doing as well as it is today. Indeed, vascular surgeons often lead in developing many of the evolving endovascular procedures that are currently the standard of care.

Yet this speech, like the one two years before, was greeted as far-fetched and wrong-headed by many of the vascular leaders of the day—certainly by the older ones. But no matter. Here it is twenty-six years later and up to 80–95 percent of all vascular lesions are or will be best treated by endovascular means, though some vascular patients still require open operations.

In 1999, another one of our most important papers, entitled "Endovascular repair of ruptured aorto-iliac aneurysms," was published in the *Journal of the American College of Surgeons* (*JACS*). In it, we presented our study of twelve high risk ruptured AAAs, in patients who were impossible to treat by open repair. All had their AAA successfully excluded by our surgeon-made EVG. Of the twelve patients, ten survived and only two died—a remarkably low 17 percent thirty-day mortality. Everybody thought we were out of our minds. They opined that what we should be doing was the standard open operation. This consisted of opening the abdomen and quickly putting a clamp on the aorta proximal to the AAA. This could be done either high in the abdomen or just below the arteries to the kidneys. A standard prosthetic vascular graft could then be sewn in to exclude the ruptured aneurysm. However, such a standard open operation could not be done in these twelve patients for various reasons. Yet ten of these twelve patients survived their EVG repair or EVAR of their ruptured AAA. I thought the value of EVAR for ruptured AAAs was proven. However, once again it took over twenty years for that to be widely accepted.

In subsequent work we found and published other important facts in the treatment of ruptured AAAs. For example, it was always thought that rapid clamping of the aorta was essential in the treatment of ruptured AAAs to prevent the patients from bleeding to death from the hole in their ruptured AAA. If this were true, there may not be enough time to carry out an EVG repair. However, what we found was that by restricting fluid resuscitation for their blood loss and allowing the patient's blood pressure to drop, most of the patients stopped bleeding long enough to undergo an EVAR. We called this aggressive fluid restriction "hypotensive hemostasis," and it worked in most (about 75 percent) of cases.

When it did not work, we alternatively developed a system for inserting a balloon catheter in the supra-celiac or upper-abdominal aorta to stop the bleeding. With the balloon in place, we also had a system for deploying the EVG and completing the EVAR successfully. This somewhat complex system was detailed in a movie I presented at the SVS and an article in the *JVS* in 2013.

Nowadays, the majority of articles and talks in our field are focused on endovascular topics. Indeed, EVAR has largely become the standard of care for ruptured AAAs, provided one has the skills and equipment to do it. However, some old-time surgeons might still call this belief heresy. Why? In my opinion it was simply their old lingering bias.

What about the present status of EVGs for the treatment of elective AAAs and other vascular lesions?

In 1995, I was asked to chair an ad hoc endovascular graft committee of the joint council of the SVS and the International Society for Cardiovascular Surgery, North American Chapter, in collaboration with the Society of Cardiovascular and Interventional Radiology and with representation from the FDA and the National Heart Lung and Blood Institute of the National Institutes of Health. This committee was charged with writing guidelines for the development and use of transluminally placed endovascular prosthetic grafts in the arterial system. I was the first of seventeen multi-specialty authors on the resulting guidelines, which were published in two prestigious journals: the *Journal of Vascular Surgery* and the *Journal of Vascular and Interventional Radiology*. I also did most of the writing work on these authoritative guidelines, which influenced EVG development and use for over a decade.

Now the field of EVGs has exploded far beyond the expectations and even the dreams of any of the authors of these guidelines. Today over 80 percent of elective AAAs being treated undergo EVAR with a procedural mortality less than 2 percent. Currently, industry-made EVGs have almost totally replaced the surgeon-made devices developed by us and the other pioneers. Even though our primitive devices worked remarkably well, industrial device makers have made EVG systems that are better, easier to use, and more versatile. Improvements in EVGs and their delivery systems are appearing with regularity for the treatment of AAAs and almost all other lesions throughout the vascular tree. Industry-made EVGs are now available to treat lesions in arteries as large as the ascending aorta (up to 4 cm in diameter) and as small as coronary or renal arteries (4 mm in diameter). Branched and fenestrated EVGs have improved the treatment of aortic aneurysms and dissections at all levels. Every operating room and angiography lab has a stock of EVGs for treating vascular emergencies and mishaps. The vascular world has changed.

Looking back, it is hard to believe how our (Marin's and mine) and Parodi's primitive surgeon-made EVGs have led to a transformation in the way most vascular lesions are treated today, and will be treated in the future. Our early work and innovation has truly been a game-changer in every sense of the word. And the game is continuing to change with better, more versatile EVGs. Millions of patients around the world will benefit as a result.

PREVENTION AND CONSERVATIVE TREATMENT IN VASCULAR DISEASE

What about preventative measures and conservative treatment in vascular disease? I also believe generally in the great value of preventative medicine. Toward that end, as a treatment for the prevention or control of vascular disease, I have been a strong advocate for statin drugs, as, among many benefits, they lower LDL cholesterol and decrease the rate of strokes, heart attacks, and death from the complications of arteriosclerosis

So how can you argue with taking a drug that makes you live longer? To me, it's a no-brainer and I myself take statins. In November 2013, the *New York Times* published an op-ed by two respected cardiologists who spoke against the wider use of statins, arguing that statins "benefit the pharmaceutical industry more than anyone else," claiming multiple nefarious side effects, even asserting that the doctors advocating statins were "conflicted." The headline blared: "Don't Give More Patients Statins."[11] I, in response, wrote a letter to the editor of the *Times*, arguing why this viewpoint was incorrect. As I stated:

> Statins are the miracle drug of our era. They have proven repeatedly and dramatically to lower the disabling and common consequences of arteriosclerosis—most prominently heart attacks, strokes and deaths. Statins avoid these vascular catastrophes not only by lowering lipids but also by a number of other beneficial effects that stabilize arterial plaques. They have minimal side effects most of which are benign. In contrast to what is implied in the Op Ed, these drugs are an easy way for people to live longer and live better, and statins cannot be replaced with a healthy life style and diet—although combining the latter with statins is a good thing.
>
> Lastly, regarding the comments about the pharmaceutical industry benefitting and physicians' conflicts of interest, both are less important than overriding patient benefit. Moreover, most statins are generic so the cost for obtaining these

---

11 John D. Abramson and Rita F. Redberg, "Don't Give More Patients Statins," *New York Times*, Nov. 13, 2013, https://www.nytimes.com/2013/11/14/opinion/dont-give-more-patients-statins.html.

miraculous drugs need not be prohibitive, and the guidelines' authors were experts who were eminently qualified to write them—despite any biases they may have.

More patients should be on statin medication. Not less!

Sadly, the *New York Times* did not publish my letter. Was this foremost newspaper biased? Of late this seems to be true in many areas—now to the point where this previously esteemed newspaper has lost much of its credibility.

What about the medical treatment or non-treatment of vascular lesions? It is definitely true that many vascular lesions are best left untreated, and many more are best treated medically by diet, drugs, and lifestyle modification. In fact, I've always preached that one should not just treat a lesion, but the entire well-being of a vascular patient. Most of the time, in patients with a small aneurysm or an asymptomatic plaque or lesion in the carotid or other vascular beds, surgery or interventional treatment is *not* needed. Sadly, many vascular specialists and other physicians do not recognize the relative benignancy of many vascular lesions.

However, these vascular specialists have a different point of view. For whatever their motivation may be, some of them hold the erroneous belief that *any* detectable lesion, particularly one causing no or mild symptoms, *should* be treated invasively by virtue of its mere existence. Metaphorically, a lesion in their minds is like a mountain that should be climbed. Why? Simply because it is there.

I believe this is totally wrong. The mere presence of a vascular lesion does not justify treatment. One motivation, of course, is the financial incentive that drives both doctors and institutions to treat (or over treat) lesions. But should one treat an asymptomatic carotid stenosis, or a femoral artery occlusion that's causing only some mild pain on walking? My belief is that most of these patients are best treated medically with reassurance, a better diet and good lipid management with statins and other drugs to control hypertension and diabetes.

Yet, as I've said again and again, medicine at both the physician and at the institutional level is often driven by the incentive of money. The whole question of ethics and motivation make it an imperfect world today in many fields—and in medicine for sure.

In fact, everything today pushes doctors to produce more RVUs (relative value units) for which they get paid, and DRGs (disease related groups) for which the hospital gets paid. Indeed, hospitals sometimes pressure doctors to perform more procedures, and occasionally threaten to pay them less if they *don't* produce enough RVUs or DRGs.

There is little compensation or financial reward for *not* invasively treating a patient. So unnecessary procedures abound in every specialty, and patients don't get the best treatment—e.g., they get procedures for asymptomatic carotid stenosis, femoral artery stents for mild or non-existent intermittent claudication (defined as leg muscle pain on walking). Sad but true. It is an imperfect world.

So, it seems that *greed* in the medical establishment has gotten worse in the last ten years. Why? As reimbursement fees for performing procedures are reduced, some doctors do more unnecessary procedures to maintain their incomes. It is a very natural human response—the way human nature works.

The most extreme case I know is a Maryland cardiologist who was charged in 2011 with falsely recording and exaggerating the presence of coronary artery blockages in patients in order to justify implanting unnecessary stents, then billing Medicare and Medicaid for these expensive procedures. (He got eight years in jail!)[12]

---

12   Mass Device Staff, "Over-stenting doc gets 8 years in jail," *MassDevice*, Nov. 14, 2011, https://www.massdevice.com/over-stenting-doc-gets-8-years-jail/.

However, most examples of physician-driven greed are much more subtle and allow poor practices to continue.

THE FUTURE OF VASCULAR SURGERY

As for the future of vascular surgery, I refer to a speech I gave in the spring of 2016, presented as a Homans Lecture of the Society for Vascular Surgery (reprinted in the Appendix). This lecture is named after John Homans, one of the most respected surgeons in the first half of the twentieth century, largely due to his seminal contributions in the treatment of venous disease.

As I stated in this lecture:

I realize that predicting the future is risky and that my predictions can be wrong. Also, as Yogi Berra said, "the future ain't what it used to be," and this applies particularly to vascular surgery because the health care system and vascular surgery's position in it has become so different from what it was. However, this topic allows me to tell you what is right and bright about American vascular surgery and the challenges it faces.

I posed the question:

What about the future for vascular surgery in ten years and beyond? What changes should we expect? What are our challenges, and how should we meet them?

First, the easy prediction. How far will the endovascular revolution go? Will all invasive treatments for vascular lesions become endovascular? It does not take a soothsayer to realize that more and more vascular lesions will become amenable to endovascular treatment. By 2026, one can predict that 75 percent to 95 percent of all vascular lesions requiring treatment will undergo an endovascular procedure. With the creativity of vascular surgeons and others, this percentage will likely increase. Moreover, all of these treatments will be deliverable via percutaneous approaches.

Does this increasing role for endovascular treatments mean that the day of open surgery is over? Definitely not. There will always be a need for hybrid (open + endovascular) repairs in 5 percent of vascular lesions. Also, there will always be a need for fully open surgery in 5 percent to 15 percent of patients requiring invasive treatment, although some of these procedures may be improved by endovascular adjuncts.

I also pointed to the value of advances in vascular surgery made possible by advances in pharmaceuticals and other technologies:

Heparin, safe contrast agents, and prosthetic vascular grafts are three prominent examples. Similarly, the explosive progress in endovascular treatments is made possible by improvements in digital imaging and the catheter-based technology our industry partners provided. Glimpses of computer-assisted three-dimensional device navigational tools are already appearing. So are systems analogous to global positioning within the vascular tree. Radiation will not be required, thereby decreasing hazards to patients and operators. Advances in robotic guidance will also decrease radiation exposure and facilitate device placement. Computer-enhanced simulation will improve training and, when patient specific, will allow procedure planning and rehearsal, thereby improving patient outcomes.

Three-dimensional printed models of lesions and blood vessels will contribute to these improvements.[13]

All in all, as I said in my Homans Lecture, the future for vascular surgery, vascular surgeons, and their patients is bright! There will be exciting new treatments, good research opportunities, and lots of patients needing our attention.

Despite some of the challenges vascular surgery faces as a specialty, I am particularly pleased that two of my granddaughters are training in vascular surgery. They chose vascular surgery because it is an ever-changing field with multiple opportunities to innovate and change patients' lives for the better. It is my hope and expectation that vascular surgery will provide them with the chance to make contributions that exceed even mine.

---

13   Veith FJ, "A look at the future of vascular surgery," John Homans Lecture of the Society for Vascular Surgery, *Journal of Vascular Surgery* 2016; 64: 885–890.

CHAPTER SIX

VALIANT CRUSADE: RECOGNIZING VASCULAR SURGERY AS AN INDEPENDENT SPECIALTY

O ne of the greatest struggles of my professional life has been in the effort to have vascular surgery recognized as a separate and independent specialty. Vascular surgeons have always been not only subordinate, they have usually been step-children to other specialties. As a result, patient well-being, the ultimate goal of specialization, suffers.

Most vascular surgeons have always wanted to be fully equal to our surgical counterparts in neurosurgery, orthopedics, urology, plastic surgery, cardiothoracic surgery, obstetrics and gynecology, otolaryngology, and ophthalmology—among the twenty-four member specialties comprising the American Board of Medical Specialties or ABMS.

But do we *have* equal independent recognition to these other specialties? No, we do not.

Instead, we are relegated to second-class status, functioning as a subspecialty within the General Surgery Board, or within institutions subservient to a department of general surgery or cardiac surgery. This should not be the case because vascular surgery fulfills all the requirements to be a separate specialty by any criterion including those of the ABMS as stated in its own bylaws.

As vascular surgeons, we have mastered highly complex surgical techniques, imaging diagnostics, and management of non-cardiac vascular disease that require an immense amount of specialized knowledge and technical skill. In addition, we have had our own specialized training programs. Yet we do not have a seat at the table when it comes to the distribution of hospital resources (i.e., equipment, space, staff, and funding) as the needs of the parent specialty always come first. Nor do we have enough training programs, which is why I and others felt it was imperative that we separate ourselves to create our own governing bodies.

But as you will read, our fight for an independent Vascular Surgery Board has been an arduous journey—filled with heartache and controversy, public debate and turf battles, and enough duplicity and vicious infighting to last a lifetime.

Over a period of eleven years, from the time of my Society for Vascular Surgery presidential address in 1996 (my first assertion that vascular surgery should be a separate specialty) until 2007, I was the most outspoken major leader in the crusade against the unfairly subordinate status of vascular surgery.

As you will see, our herculean attempts to gain our own ABMS board were contentious and created some of the most disruptive professional and personal controversies our specialty had ever witnessed. To say the least, our activism toward autonomy was deemed divisive and revolutionary by the powerful entities that opposed us.

The *New York Times* and the *Wall Street Journal*, among other media outlets, covered the public battle for separate specialty recognition in bold headlines. From within vascular surgery, the vast majority of surgeons and leaders supported our mission—until some leaders did not.

Instead, it seemed that some were seduced by institutional pressures that promised titles and rewards in exchange for standing down from our goal. Even lobbying Congress made no difference. We were up against a self-serving cartel-like structure in US-organized medicine that would not tolerate an independent vascular surgery specialty niche.

The irony is that the mission of the ABMS is to improve patient care through specialization. Yet that supposed goal became secondary to the preservation of power and the desire to control money and other resources. At all costs, our opponents wanted to maintain the status quo—the Medical Mafia at work again.

Ultimately, much to my deep disappointment, we failed to make vascular surgery a separate specialty, one of the only times I attempted to do something in my career that was not ultimately successful. In fact, the effort imploded and left me estranged from the very institution to which I had contributed so much.

In the end, the forces arrayed against us were just too powerful. Our campaign for full specialty recognition was doomed and shut down indefinitely—even though almost all other countries in the civilized world have now made vascular surgery a separate specialty!

Though I was previously accustomed to going against the grain, I never expected the deluge of critical opposition that greeted me and my colleagues in the independence effort, pushback that revealed an unusual amount of animosity within the medical establishment. But as I've learned, like any profession or business (even the healing kind), medicine is filled with backroom politics, ruthless grabs for power and duplicitous actions.

As early as the 1970s, it became apparent that committed vascular surgeons were getting consistently better outcomes and lower mortality rates than general or cardiac surgeons performing vascular surgery. That's because an ever-increasing number of more complicated open surgical procedures and other treatments were being employed, all requiring mastery of technical skill and additional knowledge that other surgeons often did not possess.

Simply put, vascular surgeons were significantly better than general surgeons at complex and risky operations involving the body's major blood vessels. In my view, most of the generalists were mere dabblers, performing vascular surgery as a part-time adjunct to a busy surgical practice in another field.

Yes, the general and cardiac surgeons wanted the rewards of doing the vascular procedures as part of their overall portfolios. Yes, they could technically *do* the procedures. But they simply couldn't perform all the demanding operations on blood vessels as well as committed vascular surgeon specialists could. Vascular patients paid the price.

So, it was a matter of competence vs. super-competence, two classes of surgeons vying for the same pool of patients.

To put it even more bluntly, many general surgeons had relatively poor knowledge of the natural history of vascular disease. Regrettably, they performed some unnecessarily invasive procedures when a conservative approach would have been best for relatively benign vascular lesions. Indeed, no treatment was often best.

Yet as surgeons, in institutions we are frequently evaluated on the number of operations performed rather than on the quality of the results. Long lengths of stay in the hospital and readmissions are thought to be marks of poor care and disadvantageous to a hospital's bottom line. So unneeded operations on less severe disease are more financially rewarding to a hospital than complex procedures with long hospital stays on patients who really need the limb or lifesaving surgery. Thus, financially driven criteria for patient treatment are sometimes the antithesis of good care in vascular surgery. Obviously, some patients require longer stays in the hospital and even readmissions to achieve optimal results.

By the early 2000s, the revolutionary introduction and rapid evolution of endovascular treatments for many vascular lesions required vascular surgeons to acquire an even greater fund of knowledge and new technical skills necessitating additional training.

Without doubt, vascular surgeons who devote their entire practice to perfecting operations and endovascular interventions that address vascular diseases should be recognized as separate specialists in their own field. It will result in better care for patients.

Moreover, as the endovascular revolution became dominant, it was clear to me that this evolutionary development in our field would clearly differentiate vascular surgery from its general surgery and cardiothoracic surgery ancestors. Indeed, the superiority of our abilities and the benefits to patients were obvious and documented in a number of scientific articles.

To put it another way, it seemed obvious to me that what *we* do is as life-altering as an orthopedist, a cardiac surgeon, a neurosurgeon, a gynecologist, a urologist, or a plastic surgeon. Yet those practitioners all have the imprimatur of being a specialty whereas we do not. The intrinsic unfairness of this seemed stunning.

But as I've stated, there was mighty resistance to this logical point of view. Indeed, the machinations of our opponents were fueled by political and economic motives, reflecting all the negative qualities of human nature when it comes to power, control, money, and prestige.

Back in the early nineties, as a relatively junior member of the SVS leadership, I was asked to negotiate with the American Board of Surgery (ABS) to see if we could get a vascular surgeon on the Residency Review Committee in Surgery (RRC-S), a group linked to the ABS that controlled the training of general and vascular surgeons.

"Don't worry, it's done," I was assured by the chairman of the ABS. But six months later, he came back and said, "It didn't happen because the directors of *my* board didn't approve it."

I had been tricked. It was apparent that the interests of general surgery were going to be served in preference to those of vascular surgery. The result was that many vascular surgery services like my own would be ill-served, because general surgery training was deemed more important than that of the vascular surgery trainees.

This friction between the two specialties was going to be a chronic problem in our continuing quest for independence. The ABS, largely dominated by its general surgery directors, was never going to put the interests of vascular surgery first. They never did.

I was personally the recipient of such injustice in the early 1990s when my vascular surgery training program was put on probation because we didn't do an adequate number of open aorto-femoral bypasses for obstructed major arteries in the abdomen. The reason we didn't do them was simple: We could treat these conditions more effectively by using the far safer and lesser procedures of percutaneous balloon angioplasty and stents. Unfortunately for me, these endovascular procedures were not yet accepted by most general and vascular surgeons. They certainly were not by the ABS and its associated RRC-S that was evaluating my training program. Several years later these endovascular procedures became the standard of care for almost all such lesions. Yet our superior and forward-looking patient care had been rewarded by unjust probation of my training program.

This was just one of the times our vascular surgery division was treated unfairly. I had other situations at Montefiore where the chairman of surgery would not even allow my vascular surgery fellows to gain credit for the cases they performed. He wanted to transfer credit for those cases to one of his general surgery residents, even though they did not perform the procedure! Why would the chairman do such a thing? Because he would look better in the eyes of his peers in general surgery? It did not seem to matter to him that this behavior smacked of dishonesty and fraudulence. Such incidents were representative of the unfairness perpetrated on vascular surgery training programs.

In any case, it was apparent to me in 1996 that vascular surgery had evolved to the point that it fulfilled all the ABMS requirements to become a new separate specialty as stated in the bylaws of that organization.

According to those bylaws, a medical specialty was defined as a group of individual doctors of medicine who, as a result of specialized effort and training in a defined field, have a high degree of similarity in their possession of a special, distinct body of scientific medical knowledge and technical ability that is not possessed in full by other specialists. These specialists concentrate their practice in the well-defined and distinct area of their special knowledge and technical ability, and they have the capacity to reproduce themselves through recognized residency training programs with a defined curriculum and specified case and procedural experiences. We checked every box.

So, in 1996, when I was president of the Society for Vascular Surgery, I highlighted the need for vascular surgery, as it evolves, to be recognized as an independent specialty by making it a prominent conclusion of my presidential address, "Charles Darwin & Vascular Surgery," which we discussed in the last chapter and which is reprinted in its entirety in the Appendix.

Among other points, I also recommended that vascular surgery had to become separate from the dominance of general surgery *administratively*. Only in this way could our own interests not be subordinated to those of general surgery on the national level (with regard to training and examinations), and locally within hospitals and medical schools.

Not surprisingly, my presidential address was regarded as heretical to the medical establishment (i.e., to the ABMS and its member boards). Etched in stone was the older tradition that vascular surgeons were subordinate to general surgeons, our so-called superiors. It did not matter that patients would be better served if vascular surgery were a separate specialty. It only mattered that the power and control of general surgery be maintained, and that all general surgeons including some poorly trained in vascular surgery be enabled to deliver sometimes inferior patient care.

The implication of my address was damning: even though general surgeons considered themselves competent in vascular surgery, many of them actually weren't. I had the temerity to make that undiplomatic assertion, which obviously annoyed the general surgeons and the broader medical establishment.

After my address to the SVS and continuing inability to gain meaningful concessions from the ABS or RRC-S, I became even more committed to make vascular surgery a separate specialty. I initially recommended that we do this collegially, playing by ABMS rules. But it soon became apparent that that wasn't going to get us where we needed to go.

Every time my colleagues representing vascular surgery made reasonable requests for fairness regarding our interests, we were double-talked but turned down by the ABS and/or the RRC-S. They would yes us to death and then nothing would happen. It became apparent that vascular surgery would have to seek its own recognition as an approved board from the American Board of Medical Specialties (ABMS).

So, the year after my Darwin address, I formed a strong alliance with the subsequent president of the SVS, Dr. James Stanley (the author of more than 325 scientific articles and 180 chapters in surgical textbooks). We also enlisted the support of other SVS leaders and officers of other important national and regional vascular surgery societies. All together, we mounted an effort to become an independent ABMS-approved Board in vascular surgery.

First, all the national vascular surgical society officers incorporated a new organization called the American Board of Vascular Surgery (ABVS) with a board of directors representing all the national and regional vascular surgery organizations in the US and Canada. There was total unanimity amongst all that we should apply for ABMS approval.

We also had strong rank-and-file support (>80 percent) in numerous polls that we took after educating all vascular surgeons on the issues of why we should be a separate specialty with our own independent Board and RRC, and how it would benefit our patients and solve many of vascular surgery's problems. Indeed, all the regional and national societies, the program directors, and every vascular surgery organization in the country supported our quest.[14]

The ABMS application, of which I was the principal author, documented that our specialty fulfilled literally all the requirements of the ABMS for obtaining a new separate ABMS approved Board, as stated in their bylaws. This application also included a provision for some general and cardiothoracic surgeons (if they were proficient in vascular surgery) to become certified in vascular surgery by documenting their commitment, clinical experience and proven acceptable results.

As the principal writer of the application, it was for me a torturous process of research, clinical data collection and getting the opinions of many others that began in 1997 and culminated in 2002. At that time, we submitted the application to petition the Liaison Committee for Specialty Boards of the ABMS. The application, which went through dozens of drafts, was a huge amount of work, showing in excruciating detail how each ABMS criterion had been fulfilled. (By this point, I had become so familiar with the bylaws of the ABMS that I knew them virtually by heart!) The finished application was endorsed by North America's thirteen major vascular surgery societies, demonstrating clearly and conclusively why vascular surgery met all the ABMS requirements to qualify for separate approved board status.

14 Veith FJ, Stanley JC, "Vascular Surgery's Identity," *Journal of Vascular Surgery* 2020; 72: 293–297. See also footnote 18.

Not least controversial, our application proved that when vascular operations were performed by surgeons who did them infrequently, the results were worse and the operative mortality higher. It was indisputable that specialization was better for patient care. That is the entire premise of the ABMS, and the one they deviated from when they rejected our application.

Shockingly, though we fulfilled all the bylaws' requirements to be an independent specialty, our ABMS application was rejected with no explanation whatsoever as to what specific criteria had not been met.[15]

When we went to lobby Congress, asking them to investigate the ABMS, a top legislative assistant of one of the senators called the president of the ABMS to ask why our application was rejected. His answer as heard by several of our lobbying group on a speaker phone, was, "I don't know. We don't keep any records related to that question."

The decision makers were not even required to spell out their reasons for rejecting a new board application. Nobody had to explain anything! The ABMS was comporting itself like a cartel. Clearly, it was an old boys' club (the Medical Mafia), and we weren't being invited into it.

Even other vascular surgeons did not always come to the rescue. Yes, the vast majority of them supported the struggle to obtain an independent vascular surgery board, though there were several elderly leaders who opposed us, as they either held positions in general surgery or aspired to such positions. These opposing individuals within vascular surgery were motivated in various ways by their general surgery colleagues to oppose our initiative and maintain the

---

15　See footnotes 14 and 18.

status quo. Often they were rewarded by positions in organizations outside vascular surgery.

For a while around the time of our application's submission, we had an overwhelming majority of support within the executive councils of all vascular surgical organizations as well as among all vascular surgeons. However, our opponents picked away at this support and persuaded, by various means, some of the emerging leaders in our specialty to join the opposition. Sadly, with a change of SVS officers in 2007, we lost the unanimity of support in the leadership of the SVS and some of the other major vascular surgical organizations. As a result, we lost control of the SVS executive committee, and that organization withdrew its support of the ABVS. In its place an SVS committee was established to deal with the independence issue. That committee never met and took no action to change the status quo.

It seemed to those of us who had mounted a great effort to have vascular surgery recognized as a separate specialty that we had lost out undemocratically to a few individuals who were vascular surgeons, but who were representing interests other than those of vascular surgery. Moreover, it seemed that our opponents had cleverly placed these individuals in positions of leadership as their agents to derail the independence initiative. And they had succeeded in doing so.

In support of this premise, in early 2003 I was contacted by a high executive of the American Board of Surgery (ABS), who told me that if I would cease my intense efforts in support of vascular surgery's independence, I would be "duly honored and suitably rewarded for the rest of my career." I failed to ask him what these rewards might be, but I assumed it would be some prominent leadership position in an important general surgery organization.

So, I asked him, if I could convince the other twenty-nine members of our ABVS board that we should lessen our efforts toward independence, what was the ABS prepared to offer us in terms of a compromise? And his answer was very simple: "Nothing." (My wife Carol was listening to this conversation on the speaker phone and remembers it well.)

"I guess this conversation is over," I told him.

And his retort? "If you ever repeat this to anyone, I will deny it." It was like something right out of *The Godfather*! That was the end of my communication with him.

Long story short, in the fall of 2004, notwithstanding inducements that were offered to the ABVS leaders to stop our support for independence, we prepared our worthy appeal to the ABMS. We filed it in February 2005. At just that moment, we got some great publicity when the *New York Times* published an article about our crusade, titled "Vascular Surgeons Bang on the Specialists' Door."[16] As they wrote:

> He would seem an unlikely radical, but Dr. Frank J. Veith is waging an aggressive and unusually public fight in the clubby world of the medical profession.
>
> A 73-year-old vascular surgeon who is the vice chairman of surgery at Montefiore Medical Center and Albert Einstein College of Medicine, in the Bronx, Dr. Veith is on a crusade aimed at the way the medical establishment divides its turf among different specialists. He and his supporters want to

---

16 Reed Abelson, "Vascular Surgeons Bang on the Specialists' Door," *New York Times*, February 11, 2005, https://www.nytimes.com/2005/02/11/health/vascular-surgeons-bang-on-the-specialists-door.html.

have vascular surgeons, doctors who operate on blood vessels, officially recognized as board-certified specialists [by a separate independent board].

Surgeons like Dr. Veith argue that this designation would improve patient care by ensuring that doctors who repair aortic aneurysms or perform other vascular surgeries are trained in that specialty. But those who oppose creation of the independent medical board that would oversee and certify that specialty say Dr. Veith and his backers are engaged in a power grab that would only fragment the field of surgery.

Either way, no one disputes the power of board certification, which is often an essential credential for doctors seeking hospital privileges. It can also be a vital marketing tool in attracting patients.

Turned down two years ago, Dr. Veith is appealing the decision today before members of a special committee of the American Medical Association and American Board of Medical Specialties, an umbrella group of the 24 existing medical boards.

I was heartened when the article stated: "Dr. Veith and others who support his effort insist that vascular surgeons are significantly better than general surgeons at complex and risky operations involving the body's major blood vessels. And an independent board of such specialists, they say, can best oversee the training of other vascular surgeons and determining the requirements for becoming a specialist."

This was music to my ears. But to maintain editorial balance, the *Times* also quoted Dr. Steven H. Miller (then the executive VP of the American Board of Medical Specialties) stating that he would "jump at the chance to make a new specialty" *if* one was needed. But he and his cronies argued that a new vascular board was unnecessary because vascular surgeons were already awarded a *subspecialty* certificate through the American Board of Surgery. Why wasn't this enough?

Indeed, almost immediately after the *New York Times* article appeared, the American Board of Surgery gave us a token sub-board in vascular surgery. But that status gave us no decision-making or operational authority over matters involving our specialty.

Our effort to pursue an independent board was diminished and then put on hold. We've been that way now for more than thirteen years because few have taken on the risks of a leadership role. Regrettably, the vascular surgery rank and file are now uninformed about the value that an independent board would have to both their patients and to themselves.

I must say that the strategies of the medical establishment to keep vascular surgery subordinate have worked extremely well: (1) delay our quest for independence with endless bureaucratic hoops and false promises, 2) delay our quest further with small, relatively meaningless concessions (like a primary certificate and a sub-board or Vascular Surgery Board within the ABS—with no operational authority), and 3) place negatively inclined vascular surgeons in leadership positions in important vascular surgical societies.

Yet some vascular surgery leaders really did believe that the primary specialty certificate was a big victory. I called it the booby prize, a relatively minor concession and a means to keep us subordinate. Yes, our specialty received some improved training paradigms, but the toxic status quo was maintained, with vascular surgery remaining subordinate and subservient within institutions and to the directors of the ABS and its associated residency review committee.

And though there is a non-independent board of vascular surgery, which is called the Vascular Surgery Board of the ABS, some members of that board have their allegiance to general surgery. That board takes care of the menial details, but it doesn't have any operational or executive authority over most of the critical and important issues pertaining to vascular surgery.

Many in our field argued that the training of general surgeons and vascular surgeons needed to be handled by one body. I strenuously disagreed, arguing that vascular surgical operations and education in their training were being wasted on generalists who were either unlikely to ever again perform major vascular operations or who may fool themselves into thinking they can handle such cases which could unexpectedly turn complicated.

Despite a strong showing in the public arena (both the *New York Times* piece and another even more supportive article in the *Wall Street Journal*[17]), we were defeated.

It was the perfect storm turned against us, driven by the loss of support within the SVS in 2007, the rejection of our application by the ABMS, and the denial of its appeal—again with no reason given for the denial. Once again, the powerful and unaccountable old-boys' club of the cartel-like ABMS and its member boards had triumphed over a justified progressive change that would have helped patients receive better care.

Clearly, the common good was not their goal. Instead, deception and playing dirty defined the rules of the game. We tried to play by the rules and be conciliatory, but the opposition was deceptive and totally

---

17 Thomas M. Burton, "The Surgery Your Doctor Shouldn't Perform: Vascular Procedure Carries Greater Risks When Done By General Surgeons," *Wall Street Journal*, December 30, 2003.

uncompromising. Indeed, even in the aftermath of our defeat, those who supported independence (like me) were treated as troublemakers and sometimes harmed for their efforts. More on that in a moment.

This entire shameful process is well documented in a 2016 article in the *Annals of Vascular Surgery*.[18] The article and the accompanying documentary appendices took up an entire issue of the publication. It clearly demonstrated just how unfair and self-serving organized medicine can be in the United States.

The application and appeals process for us to obtain an ABMS approved independent vascular surgery board was, at the time, a kangaroo court. Clearly, the all-powerful American Board of Medical Specialties and its member boards seemed to be in bed together, allied against making vascular surgery a separate specialty. From the outset we were doomed to failure, as I had been forewarned by a friendly member of the ABMS before starting our effort. I didn't believe him then, but sadly he was right.

After our appeal was rejected, the *New York Times* did a follow-up piece on March 18, 2005. It was titled "New Board For Surgeons Denied Again."[19] They reported that the appeals panel for the committee said it found no evidence of bias, claiming that both sides received what they called "a fair and equitable hearing."

Obviously this was wrong, but I was not surprised to read that many doctors who opposed the new board said it was unnecessary:

---

18 Stanley JC, Veith FJ, "The American Board of Vascular Surgery and Independence of the Specialty," *Annals of Vascular Surgery* 2016; 37: 3–331. See also footnote 14.

19 Reed Abelson, "New Board for Surgeons Denied Again," *New York Times*, March 18, 2005, https://www.nytimes.com/2005/03/18/business/new-board-for-surgeons-denied-again.html.

Dr. Veith says he and his colleagues are now considering their options, which include submitting another application, creating a medical board outside the umbrella group or lobbying Congress for some sort of governmental action.

"We haven't made a final decision," he said. "The one thing we're not going to do is quit."

Having been treated so unfairly, we did consider our legal options. It was during this time that we approached a high-powered New York attorney, Oliver Koppell, and discussed with him the option of filing a class action lawsuit against the ABMS. Koppell thought we had a good chance to win. In fact, armed with the unanimous support of thirty directors of the ABVS board, we were about to proceed with it.

However, when some of our opponents found out about our intention to file the lawsuit, they threatened to counter sue the ABVS officers personally. At the time, I was out of the country, on a two-week trip to New Zealand as a visiting professor. In my absence, enormous pressure was brought to bear on my ABVS vice chairman (Dr. Robert Hobson), who was urged to drop the suit.

Although I had instructed Koppell to file the lawsuit before I left on the trip, my vice chairman and others succumbed to the pressure and threats and prevented that filing. By the time I returned from New Zealand, I found out that the lawsuit had been abandoned. And that was that. While I was subsequently punished for my advocacy of vascular surgery independence, those vascular surgeons who had withdrawn support of the ABVS were the recipients of the largesse of the all-powerful medical establishment. Some became directors of the ABS, others were chosen president of a regional surgical society, others were appointed to prestigious chairs of general surgery departments or deans of medical schools.

In the end, the medical establishment had proven that it had the muscle to defeat us. And so it remains to this day, even though vascular surgery in most hospitals and institutions still suffers from its status as a subordinate and often subservient subspecialty.

The result of this is that we're not able to train as many surgeons as we would like to. It's a very complex problem. And in my opinion, we need now more than ever an independent board so that we can help to define and brand vascular surgery as the specialty it is, which is the specialty solely devoted to taking care of non-cardiac vascular disease patients.

To this day, some prominent vascular surgeons do not regard this as an important issue. This is possibly because their "ox isn't getting gored" at the present time. My greatest fear is that vascular surgery as a discipline will be usurped or weakened in large part by interventional cardiology. While some cardiologists are innovative thought leaders and do what they do brilliantly, some others just tack on vascular disease patients as an add-on to their cardiac practice. The ultimate loser in this is, of course, the vascular surgeons, but more importantly, the patients whom we serve, because they are the ones sometimes getting hurt by substandard or unnecessary care.

By the time our appeal was rejected in 2005, I had alienated a great number of people at the top tiers of the ABS, the ABMS, and even the AMA. The fallout for me wasn't pleasant.

After a thirty-year career at Montefiore, I was forced out or terminated as a full-time staff member at the end of 2005. No reason was given then. However, I found out later that my termination was the result of my leadership efforts to establish a new independent specialty.

As I learned in 2007, someone on the Accreditation Council for Graduate Medical Education (ACGME), the parent body of residency review committees, called a Montefiore trustee to tell them to "get rid of Frank Veith because he is causing trouble for the ABMS by exposing their bad behavior."

I heard about this revengeful persuasive phone call from two reliable sources connected to the ACGME, but I couldn't prove it because I had no written evidence. So, I chose not to fight my termination legally, especially since one of my sources died before he could be deposed.

Even though I knew the backstory, I was never actually told by Montefiore why I was terminated. It certainly was not because of any decrease in revenue. I still was sought out by many patients, and I ran my annual VEITHsymposium, which was financially rewarding for Montefiore. Not to mention the obvious, that I was still a surgeon with exceptional results and an excellent reputation.

Thus my termination was entirely political. Moreover, Montefiore's president did not defend me because I had respectfully disagreed with him on multiple issues. One of those issues was my declining his request to take additional responsibility for cardiac surgery (a group of surgeons with conflicting priorities) when I was the chairman of surgery. Another issue was my telling the president that a cardiac surgery chairman candidate who was well known academically would not be able to establish a large referral cardiac surgery practice in the inner-city Bronx. The president hired the cardiac surgeon as department head anyhow. As I had predicted, he was unable to establish a substantial referral practice because there were more prestigious cardiac surgery departments at Manhattan hospitals. The president never forgave me for giving him the correct advice.

Still another source of disagreement was when the Montefiore leadership took control of my service so they could hire some vascular surgeons who increased hospital revenues by doing questionably indicated procedures. This was a calculated move that I opposed vehemently. But those surgeons were hired anyhow, for big salaries.

Leaving my medical home of thirty-eight years at age seventy-three was painful, yes. I felt badly at first. Rejection is a bitter pill to swallow.

Many of my colleagues knew what was happening and tried to help, but they really couldn't. My wife, Carol, was incredibly supportive, saying leaving Montefiore with all its stresses was the best thing that could possibly happen to me and opened new opportunities. She was right as I bounced back quickly. My family and wide circle of friends around the world were also supportive, which helped a lot to overcome the injustice of my Montefiore termination. I realize now that institutional appreciation for years of good work and loyalty is a rare commodity, as I have seen other high-achieving vascular surgeons disrespected and quickly forgotten once they get fired, older or retire.

However, this unpleasant termination made me see more clearly than ever that I was living in an imperfect medical world, peopled by some corrupt and self-serving administrators who put money over quality with little or no institutional loyalty to good doctors. It also confirmed my belief that greed, jealousy, and self-gain were powerful motivators of human behavior. In fact, in my view, these motivators often extend beyond medicine to all professions, to businesses, and to political leaders. There remains too little concern in the US today for ethics, fairness, altruism, or pursuing the greater good.

In my 2016 John Homans Lecture to the SVS, I spoke and wrote about this state of things today generally and in the health care system:

> We live in an imperfect world. We see it in our political leaders who are owned by special interests. We see it in many lawyers who want to translate every untoward effect or bad outcome into a compensatory judgment, with a large share for themselves. We see it in Wall Street and insurance companies that place profit above all else. And yes, we see it in our health care system, in which doctors are able to perform unnecessary procedures for financial gain.
>
> The overuse of outpatient vein centers by those who are not even vascular specialists is only one example. More importantly, institutional leaders view everything through their prism of diagnosis-related groups (DRGs, by which hospitals get paid), relative value units (RVUs, by which doctors are reimbursed), and dollars. Quality care and appropriate care are totally overshadowed by the need to generate money, and poor or unnecessary care is tolerated if providers bring in the patients, the RVUs, and the dollars. There is no easy solution, but clearly, we need an ethical revolution in our country and a return to old-style moral values and behavior. How to do this or how to solve other problems in the US health care system are challenges beyond the scope of this discussion.

I had helped transform a second-rate institution in the indigent provinces of the Bronx with a self-serving institutional leadership and administration that valued money and control over excellence. But I had made Montefiore well known and esteemed with our pioneering research and outstanding surgical accomplishments.

What had they done for me other than exploit my accomplishments for fundraising purposes and then pay me poorly? Not so much.[20] Their betrayal was positively Shakespearean.

Admittedly, I didn't learn how to deal with career adversity until fairly late in my career. But adversity is omnipresent in life, and everyone will face it sooner or later. Sometimes it comes in the form of being fired from a job, which can be very demoralizing. The natural human tendency is to react intensely—to fight the inevitable, or to try to get even, which is always a bad mistake.

But as I've learned, how you deal with adversity will inevitably determine your future successes. If you get fired, try not to overreact. Your firing might be unfair, it might be due to jealousy or a crazy boss. But what is the point of fighting back with lawsuits? It's expensive and makes the lawyers rich. The best revenge is finding a better job, and gaining future success. I can tell you that getting terminated did not hurt my career at all. In fact, making Montefiore famous had enhanced my reputation. Leaving the institution was the best thing that could have happened to me, a great relief and benefit to my psyche. It was like escaping from a gulag. After just a few months, everything changed when I was given new positions at far better institutions—New York University (NYU) and the Cleveland Clinic—where I was much better appreciated and respected. At both institutions, I would thereafter be engaged in teaching and

---

20 In 1995, only when I received two excellent leadership job offers from Columbia and Mount Sinai did Montefiore give me control of my own service and raise my salary in an effort to keep me at the hospital. I agreed to stay, but only for five years, which I thought would be enough to get me to seventy. It was a bad bargain. After five years, things went back to the usual unscrupulous jungle-like behavior that was typical of Montefiore and many other medical institutions.

mentoring young doctors. At the Cleveland Clinic, a chair was established for me (the William J. von Liebig Chair in Vascular Surgery) in 2006. Then, in 2013 at NYU, the Frank J. Veith Chair in Vascular and Endovascular Surgery was also created. I was elated!

Talk about turning lemons into lemonade: as I always say, the best revenge when you're wronged is to succeed in your subsequent ventures.[21]

And succeed I did. I also now had full ownership of the VEITHsymposium, the subject of the next chapter.

I am sometimes asked, "When do you intend to retire?" Never! From 1964 to the present, I have never stopped working, treating patients, and always mentoring, teaching, writing and publishing, and of course, leading the VEITHsymposium, which has become an ever more demanding and rewarding job as the meeting has gained importance and grown in size.

As for the future of vascular surgery, it is going to survive. However, I am concerned that unless we do a better job of establishing our identity and gaining specialty status, we will survive in a diminished form. Most troubling is the trend that other specialties will continue to control our resources—which invariably go to the parent specialty whenever there is a conflict of interest.

---

21 I should explain that I had obtained funding for a Liebig Chair at Montefiore with a contract that I would hold that chair as long as I was professionally active. The agreement to that effect was signed by Montefiore's president. Of course, they violated that agreement once they terminated me—even though they had been gifted $3 million for the chair. Neither I nor the Liebig Foundation chose to take legal action. It was my belief that it would have been costly and emotionally consuming. The Liebig Foundation did establish a second Liebig Chair for me at the Cleveland Clinic—albeit without funding.

As I stated in my 2016 Homans lecture: "To survive, vascular surgery needs to unify, recognize this inequity, and fix it. This can only be done if all vascular surgeons and the SVS engage vigorously in this issue. It can also help vascular surgery brand itself as the specialty that best takes care of blood vessels and their diseases. Such branding is something vascular surgery has not done well to date."

No doubt, we must brand ourselves as the complete vascular disease physician. To lend support, the SVS and other vascular societies must mount a robust public education campaign, targeted to other physicians and to the lay public, to inform them about vascular disease, its prevention and treatment, and to let them know who and what we are. Without such a campaign, other interventional specialists will eat our lunch, as they are doing in many communities.

As an example, interventional cardiologists do a spectacular job caring for patients with heart disease. But they also are expanding their role into non-cardiac vascular disease, and they have enabling assets. Cardiologists control patients, have interventional skills and have a financial incentive to refer to one another. They are capable doctors, and they are much more numerous than vascular surgeons. They are vigorous in adding to their numbers and in expanding their treatments to areas outside the heart. Many have been heard to say publicly that they should replace vascular surgeons. Some exemplary statements include: "Vascular surgery is dead, R.I.P." and "Vascular surgeons, bend over and kiss your butt good-bye."

Therefore we should re-engage to obtain ABMS approval for specialty status. While there will be strong opposition, with unity within the specialty this opposition can be overcome. Other evolving specialties have done it. We can do it too. And by doing so, we can pave the way for a brighter future. Most importantly, as I've stated repeatedly, patients will be the ultimate beneficiaries.

Our societies could mount such a campaign, and they need leaders willing to go against the grain. Such leaders sometimes lose and die professionally. I lost on this issue but was fortunate enough to survive.

CHAPTER SEVEN

ALL UNDER ONE TENT: THE VEITHSYMPOSIUM

O ne of the most important achievements of my professional career has been leading the VEITHsymposium—an international medical conference for vascular surgeons, physicians of multiple specialties, and industry participants from medical device and pharmaceutical companies.

Now in its forty-ninth year, this continuing medical education (CME) symposium is considered the largest vascular meeting in the world, drawing an audience of up to five thousand attendees annually and providing an invaluable opportunity for collegial interaction and an exchange of crucial current information. It's a gigantic undertaking that takes our team an entire year to plan. The meeting's program itself fills 128 pages and features over 700 speakers who present talks on over 1,000 topics.

During this five-day event, we offer participants an in-depth, immersive experience: We share updates on the latest advances in all aspects of vascular disease management. Current pharmacologic, radiologic, surgical, and endovascular techniques, technologies and devices are presented and analyzed—along with discussions of when these treatments are justified and indicated and when they are not. Ongoing controversies are highlighted and debated. Updates on clinical trials, new concepts, and important issues are presented and discussed. All that is currently of interest and importance to a vascular surgeon or other vascular specialist is covered. The meeting is a veritable goldmine of medical knowledge, reflecting the immense growth of interest in non-cardiac vascular disease and its natural history, diagnosis, and treatments—conservative and invasive (both open and endo) and medical (drugs, diet and lifestyle). We cover everything that a vascular surgeon or specialist needs to know.

Throughout the eleven-hour days, participants are continually challenged with new data and fresh ideas in short presentations and relevant panel discussions. The formal presentations and panels are expanded on in related attendee interactions in the industry pavilions and exhibits—and in informal discussions outside the auditoriums. The impact of our meeting is felt long after the meeting as the vascular surgeons and specialists bring what they have learned not only to their own practice but also to the attention of their colleagues. Patients are the ultimate beneficiaries of all this new knowledge and the improved care it facilitates.

It is important to note that the name of our event, VEITHsymposium, has absolutely nothing to do with my last name. *VEITH* is an acronym representing: Vascular, Endovascular, Issues, Techniques, Horizons, a concept that covers all the goals our meeting is intended to fulfill. But because the name of the symposium could be confused with a personal brand, I suggested years ago that we rename the meeting, feeling that folks would think me too egocentric and self-serving to keep it. However, with the persuasion of one of our administrators, I agreed to keep it. There were also political and legal factors at play.

THE MEDICAL JUNGLE

As you have already read, I was terminated after thirty-eight years at Montefiore for my activism to make vascular surgery a specialty. By that point, I had already been leading the symposium for decades, and it had become a real success, gaining supportive corporate sponsors, a good reputation, and attracting top-notch speakers of international repute.

Understandably, Montefiore wanted to hold on to this asset even after my termination at the end of 2005, since the prestigious symposium generated a significant amount of revenue beyond its costs—revenues that I was unaware of because Montefiore maintained tight secrecy over the meeting's finances. The Montefiore brass was revenue driven and could legally claim *ownership* of the symposium because I was a full-time employee of the hospital. However, since the talented Jackie Simpson and I had done 90 percent of the work preparing the meeting's program and we had the relationship with all the speakers around the world, I felt that I should own the meeting if Montefiore and I ever parted ways. I sought legal advice and was told that Montefiore was entitled to ownership as long as I was a full-time employee. In order to strengthen any claim I might have to the meeting, I agreed to call it the VEITHsymposium and trademarked the name—despite my previous reluctance to do so.

So when I was unexpectedly terminated and Montefiore, which held the meeting's hotel contract with its financial obligations, wanted to keep the meeting, I threatened to put on a competing meeting at the same time. Montefiore was fearful of losing money if doctors came to my meeting and not theirs. So they let me take on the meeting's ownership and its financial hotel obligations. I happily agreed to do so.

As owner of the meeting, we were able to get the Cleveland Clinic to sponsor it, provide CME accreditation, and assume a major

147

share of any financial risk. So in the years after 2005, the meeting could not only continue to exist, but it was also able to grow in size and importance to a point where it has become a crucial educational event for the vascular community in the United States and around the entire world. In our last meetings before the COVID pandemic, 35–40 percent of our attendees and faculty came from Europe, South America, Asia, or Australia/New Zealand and even Africa.

The symposium started in 1969 as a small conference led by Dr. Henry Haimovici, who had been the chief of vascular surgery at Montefiore Medical Center before me.

Haimovici—also one of the founders of the International Society of Cardiovascular Surgery (ISCVS)—was a pioneer in our field, the author of ten books and over two hundred journal articles. Among his best were his groundbreaking monograph on *Metabolic Complications of Acute Arterial Occlusion and Related Conditions* (1988) and his classic textbook, *Vascular Surgery: Principles and Techniques* (1976), one of the good textbooks covering vascular surgery.

The early meetings chaired by Dr. Haimovici were held in New York's old Roosevelt Hotel—an elegant structure on East 45th Street named after President Theodore Roosevelt. Built in 1924, the hotel was known as the Grande Dame of Madison Avenue. Its antique French marble and limestone façade was impressive to all those who saw it. It was an ideal spot for a medical conference that intended to draw a prestigious group of medical superstars.

But at first, we didn't need a very big ballroom. In the early days, the meeting was a modest two-day event with about a hundred attendees and fifteen speakers, the entire line-up summarized in a two-page program.

In 1971, however, when I succeeded Dr. Haimovici as chief of the division of vascular surgery at Montefiore, I accordingly followed him as the chairman of the symposium, a role I was eager to take on. Over the next forty-five years, as the field of vascular surgery matured as a specialty, the event exploded in size. As time passed, we moved it to ever-larger hotels in Manhattan—from the Roosevelt to the Grand Hyatt, the Essex House, the Waldorf Astoria, the Marriott Marquis, the Sheraton, and ending up in New York City's biggest hotel venue, the New York Hilton Midtown.

Through it all, we always resisted the temptation to host the event at a convention center, because that would have required busing participants back and forth with the disadvantage of horrendous rush-hour traffic delays. A hotel was a warmer place to conduct a symposium, with more elegant amenities than a huge impersonal and drafty convention center.

The meeting's exponential growth, prestige, and success are based on multiple factors mixed in with some good luck.

There are, of course, many other vascular meetings out there, including a major and excellent one sponsored by the Society for Vascular Surgery (SVS). So we do not hold a monopoly on the field by any means. But we became dominant mainly because of the depth and variety of the program itself, which covered everything that was new, important, or controversial in our field. I always took great pains to highlight controversy and colliding opinions and to present all sides of burning questions.

From all these discussion topics, you can see that our team devoted themselves to creating the best, most complete program possible. But no matter how good our standard, we still needed to get the word out there in order to advertise and market the event. During the first eighteen years, as we only had one part-time PR person to help, the symposium grew mostly by word-of-mouth promotion, with the event always based in New York City.

The city itself, easily accessible to participants from all parts of the world, was always a major asset of the meeting, an obviously compelling place for participants to visit with its plethora of restaurants, museums, and cultural activities. And we always treated our faculty well—inviting them to hit Broadway shows and openings rather than keeping them trapped at boring faculty dinners. In addition, as we invited larger faculties, they usually brought along their colleagues.

We found that having the symposium in New York also contributed to drawing large numbers of out-of-US faculty attendees. These foreign participants were particularly valuable to American doctors because they kept us apprised of their newer technologies, which were often restricted or delayed in the US due to stricter FDA requirements (which demand that we demonstrate proven safety and effectiveness).

Once we were all assembled in New York, we were united in a common mission—to understand the increasing complexity and breadth of vascular surgery and multispecialty vascular disease treatment.

Remember, as you've already read, up until the early 1990s, vascular surgery had been a bit stagnant in innovation. But the endovascular revolution had transformed this lethargy, and we were among the first medical conferences to realize this and capitalize on it.

As vascular surgery grew and became largely endovascular,

there was an explosion of knowledge and new devices that vascular specialists needed to know about. This included dramatic endovascular treatments, including EVGs, as well as a plethora of new, effective techniques for using them. There were also striking advances in medical and drug treatment of vascular disease—as with statins. Our goal was to represent the totality of this ever-evolving field, covering all treatments for non-cardiac vascular disease. Doing so made our symposium a true game-changer.

In my view, staying up to date could only be accomplished by in-person attendance at a balanced, unbiased symposium such as ours. Why? Because textbooks, journals, and internet sites, though valuable, can never provide the up-to-date nuance and depth of a medical conference held in real time.

As we well know, textbooks are often five years out of date and are sometimes biased by the opinions and training of the authors and editors. And half the time, that bylined expert actually delegated the writing to a junior writer who didn't know up from down. Textbooks, in my opinion, are a breed of shrinking importance.

Journals are likewise often out of date and/or often reflect the bias of the author, the reviewers, or the editors of the journal. I am not minimizing the value of journals; they obviously offer cutting-edge scientific research. But one can't rely on them entirely.

Least reliable but most accessible, of course, is internet data, which provide facts and research that are often faulty, biased, or commercially driven—not to be trusted just because you can click on it.

All this points to the inevitable: There is no substitute for an in-person, face-to-face interactive medical conference with industry representation and participation, all of which offer up-to-date information about cutting-edge research, surgical techniques, and interventional procedures with great breadth and perspective. No other forum can duplicate this kind of multi-dimensional exposure, which is why I believe there will always be a need for medical meetings to go on in perpetuity. There is no substitute for direct human interaction in medical education, as in many other forms of human behavior.

Equally important, an in-person event allows vascular surgeons and other specialists the chance to interact with one another socially. This includes interactions between fellow doctor attendees, plus meetings with faculty and industry representatives. In fact, I would say that the interplay and socializing amongst the doctors, trainees, and industry representatives is as important as the talks themselves. This is why virtual meetings, although valuable, are not as effective.

Throughout my career, I have attended hundreds of such medical conferences and have always taken them quite seriously. I felt that I owed it to my patients to attend, watch, and listen. I have also encouraged other physicians to do the same.

Despite the thousands of participants, one unique feature of our meeting is that it runs precisely on time! How? We have dedicated ourselves to limiting speakers to what we call "short talks," presentations lasting five to six minutes each, some as short as four and a half minutes. This protocol grew out of our desire to include as many speakers as possible from different specialties and with widely divergent views.

The idea for the short talks arose when we saw television news interviews with prominent government officials and others, offering digestible sound bites that seldom lasted more than three minutes. Even in a compressed timespan, the interviewer managed to extract and encapsulate the essential points of interest. These segments whet the appetite of the audience to learn more, though some left feeling satisfied. I thought to myself, "That is a technique we can use."

When faculty members know in advance that they only have five to six minutes to speak, it forces them to prepare better and focus their remarks solely on the key points they wish to get across. They distill their talk down to the essentials, the kernel of new information at hand, eliminating content that is unnecessary or repetitive. I often joke that you could tell your entire life story in six minutes, so why can't doctors give a complex presentation in that time?

Best of all, by keeping the presentations short, we could present many opposing views on controversial topics, and provide complete coverage of all that was new and interesting in the vascular field. Airing of contrary points of views and exposing all sides of topics also brings excitement and energy to the meeting, which helps it hold the attention of even a large audience.

Additionally, keeping the talks short with many views on a single topic minimized faculty bias and provided an optimally balanced view of competing techniques and technologies.

Admittedly, creating a succinct talk isn't an easy thing to do. It requires *more* preparation to make it sing. But the end result allows more speakers to take the stage.

Keep in mind that we typically have three meetings running at the same time in adjoining rooms, so it's a logistical feat to get multiple speakers on and off right on time—yet another reason we must be militant about adhering to the time limits.

After attempting many unsuccessful and clumsy techniques to keep speakers on time, we finally arrived at a method that works and is relatively painless. We place an electronic timer icon on the corner of the speakers' slides so that the speaker and the audience can see it. A speaker can run over their time by thirty seconds. But after fifty seconds, the speaker's slides are turned off! They almost always stop thereafter. We enforce this time limit absolutely. No other meeting did so when we introduced the technique. But after our symposium pioneered this short-talk-by-experts format, other meetings around the world adopted similar methods. This allowed meetings to run precisely on schedule so attendees could reliably catch the talk they *wanted* to hear, even when there were concurrent sessions going on in several rooms. The talks stayed on time.

Our unique short talk format (a counterintuitive approach to medical conferences that typically feature laborious presentations of ten minutes up to half an hour each) has allowed VEITHsymposium to fulfill its primary vision—which is to provide a comprehensive overview of the most up-to-date, unbiased data available.

Once we earned the reputation for sticking to our time limit, it's amazing how speakers adjusted. It's Parkinson's Law—the amount of work required adjusts to the time available for its completion.

A second key feature of our symposium is meeting our industry partners—medical device and pharmaceutical company executives, marketers, inventors, and research scientists. Inviting these participants to a medical conference was traditionally considered a no-no, too commercialized for a symposium of physicians.

Yet, as we all know, industry research and development and the newest innovative technologies are crucially important for the development of medical products, which lead to better patient care. Indeed, only via a partnership between doctors and industry can the best technologies and drugs be made widely and rapidly available, leading directly to better patient care. This has become increasingly important as the endovascular revolution has progressed.

However, over the years, other conferences had typically treated industry folks like second-class citizens, unwelcome and largely marginalized or disregarded except as a source of funding. On the contrary, we were the first to recognize our industry colleagues as essential and equal partners in optimizing vascular care.

Accordingly, we treated them with the respect they deserved, and were responsive to their needs. This led directly to the pavilion concept by which we provided our industry partners with a dedicated separate space that allowed them to interact directly with their customers. They could easily demonstrate the advantages and workings of new products and develop relationships and contacts, which enabled their physician customers to optimize the use of these products in their operating rooms or angiography suites.

In short, both our pavilions and exhibit halls offered participants invaluable educational materials that ultimately led to improved patient care, while helping our industry partners market their products more effectively.

Despite the logic of creating an open dialogue between doctors and medical companies, there was always the possibility of unfair or dishonest promotion of industry's products. Such potential conflicts of interest have been raised as reasons to separate doctors from industry. Much to my regret, there's an ongoing effort by some state governments and universities to separate doctors from industry based on the potential for conflicts of interest and the abuses that have occurred.[22]

Although a few flagrant conflict of interest abuses have occurred—particularly in the area of devices for spine and orthopedic surgery—I

---

22   Aaron Mitchell and Deborah Korenstein, "Drug companies' payments and gifts affect physicians' prescribing. It's time to turn off the spigot," *Stat*, December 4, 2020. https://www.statnews.com/2020/12/04/drug-companies-payments-gifts-affect-physician-prescribing.

don't believe we should throw the baby out with the bath water. Yes, the relationship between physicians and device and pharmaceutical industries is a complicated one, and we cannot tolerate gross conflicts of interest. But these conflicts are much less common among doctors and industry than they are among elected officials and their large donors. There are mechanisms to prevent such doctor-industry abuses. Moreover, I believe the hostile atmosphere that exists toward doctor-industry relationships is overblown and misguided.

To this point, I wrote an article titled "Why the On-Going Initiative to Separate Physicians from Industry Is a Witch Hunt That Is Bad for Patients and Society."[23]

In this article, while I acknowledge that there are "flagrant abuses and excessive hidden financial rewards to doctors," there are several reasons I disagree with the initiative supported by several states (MA, VT) and universities (like Harvard, Stanford, and Michigan) to sever the relationship between industry and MDs altogether.

First, as I said, physicians and surgeons rely upon industry to create the products and technologies we need. We can't afford to do it on our own. For example, when we have an idea about a device or the need for a new drug, we need the financial resources and engineering or chemical know-how of industry in order to bring that device or medication to its optimal development and clinical fruition. This can only happen when physicians communicate their needs and industry follows through with the devices and drugs we require.

---

23   Frank J. Veith, "Why the On-Going Initiative to Separate Physicians from Industry Is a Witch Hunt That Is Bad for Patients and Society," *MedScape*, September 28, 2017, https://www.medscape.com/viewarticle/885824

Second, physicians also have the expertise to assist in the development and evaluation of effective drugs, devices, and assays.

Third, industry-sponsored medical education helps keep MDs informed about new developments, new devices, and how they should be used most safely and effectively. Sure, there is opportunity for the introduction of bias, but this can be minimized by appropriate safeguards.

At our conference, we try as hard as possible to be unbiased in our presentations on devices—presenting pro and con opinions and debates. We have an excellent reputation for being above reproach in this regard. In addition, there are Accreditation Council on Continuing Medical Education (ACCME) rules that we scrupulously follow in order to prevent the false presentation of data. In addition, our multi-faculty/short talk protocols definitely minimize the possibility of biased and unfairly conflicted presentations. And, of course, since I largely make up and am responsible for the program, I religiously do so to prevent conflicts of interest.

In addition, from a practical point of view, an educational symposium like ours depends upon financial support from industry in order to produce a wide-ranging program. Without that support, meetings for continuing medical education would be largely eliminated, and MDs would be forced to get all their continuing education on-line or from textbooks and journal articles. As stated earlier, such publications are notoriously out of date and in some cases heavily biased.

Fourth, without industry representatives to enlighten vascular specialists in the use and pitfalls of individual devices, our learning process would be more difficult and dangerous to patients. Indeed, some industry representatives have far more familiarity with their devices than the physician and surgeon specialists who are using them either initially or sporadically. The result of these representatives' participation is that patients are cared for better and more safely.

Fifth, industry-sponsored courses on these devices help doctors learn to use them better and more safely, and industry-sponsored support of training for vascular residents almost always has positive effects for patients and the trainees.

In short, with all these educational advantages, we need to strongly support preserving the positive aspects of the natural relationships between doctors and industry. Maintaining such relationships is one of the hallmarks of the VEITHsymposium that will endure.

Another key feature of VEITHsymposium is the availability of a library that captures all our speakers and panels—the talks, slides, and group discussions, indexed by topic and presenter.

This invaluable library, which is enabled by recent advances in computer technology, memorializes the meeting and makes it possible for attendees to view and hear parts of it that they may have missed or want to review again later on. It is a unique resource that provides a current overview of the state of the vascular art. It can be used for teaching, review, patient management, and as a guide to the literature. The library is also available to those who cannot attend our meeting and to our industry partners as well.

Among the compelling topics we've covered recently: Advances in parallel EVGs in which the branch graft is placed entirely outside the main graft rather than through a hole in it and how these parallel grafts compare with branched and fenestrated EVGs in which the branches go through holes in the main graft. These are very controversial topics provoking much interest. So also are the sessions on advances in the treatment of lower-extremity ischemia with emerging information on new endovascular technologies and techniques for treating especially distal disease in the ankle and foot regions. There are also exciting sessions on evolving carotid treatment, improvements in carotid artery stenting, and aortic dissections. There is also an abundance of new and useful information at the expanded venous sessions and those devoted to stroke treatments and prophylaxis, arteriovenous access, and arteriovenous malformations. The library is linked directly to our program, making it easy to search. It reproduces all the formal parts of the entire meeting except for the vitally important personal interactions and presentations in the industry pavilions, the exhibit halls and elsewhere informally between individual attendees.

An additional innovative feature of our meeting has been the introduction of the Associate Faculty Program, which affords younger, less well-known practicing vascular surgeons and trainees the opportunity to present their ongoing clinical research and experience. Although the idea of inviting a younger generation of physicians to speak sounds like a no-brainer, we were actually one of the first major medical conferences to do so, an innovation since copied by many.

Previously, symposiums focused almost exclusively on booking senior faculty members with recognized names and established reputations. Yet we discovered that some of the best ideas come from younger people. Moreover, giving younger physicians a time slot on the program is a great opportunity for them to gain valuable podium speaking experience while publicly highlighting their work.

The creation of this program not only reflects our commitment to junior faculty, but it also allows our program to have unlimited inclusivity since any vascular specialist/surgeon can submit an abstract that will almost certainly be accepted for presentation. In addition, this program allows younger, less well-known physicians to get their work cited in a journal. Abstracts presented at the symposium are usually published in an online supplement to the *Journal of Vascular Surgery.*

Finally, we introduced an additional VEITHsymposium hallmark when we were the first vascular surgery organization to bring together physicians of multiple disciplines in the interest of providing new information and improving patient care.

We are, in fact, eager to recognize the contributions of other specialties and specialists. This includes recognizing the importance of interventional cardiologists, interventional radiologists and vascular medicine experts in the field and inviting them to be on our faculty—which has been especially important as the endovascular revolution has progressed. We welcome not only interventional vascular experts but also radiologists, cardiologists, and others whose work bears on vascular disease and its treatment. The result is a spirited and informative exchange of clinical experience and scientific innovation, which allows members of each specialty to profit from learning the unique skills and approaches of other specialties, thereby improving their ability to care for vascular patients.

Building on this idea of inclusion, our intent for the future is to make our meeting even more multi-specialty than it already has been. (Up until this time, 25 percent of our speakers derive from specialties other than vascular surgery.) Going forward, we will add a greater percentage of experts in other specialties to our leadership team in order to further develop our programs.

By doing this, we will hopefully attract more non-vascular surgeon attendees, who can benefit enormously from the voluminous amount of information presented at the symposium, perspectives and advances that they cannot acquire at their own specialty meetings. As I always say, the beauty of the VEITHsymposium is that everything vascular is all under one tent!

There have been some wonderful memories of our symposium over the course of decades. For example, in 1992 we invited Dr. Parodi to speak. Back then, as you've already read, he was an unknown South American vascular surgeon, eager to present his early work on EVAR in the US. Appearing at our meeting bestowed on him the credibility and recognition he deserved. Back then, no one in vascular surgery paid much heed to endovascular procedures.

That was the year we enticed him to come to New York by offering him a prominent spot on our meeting's program. In turn, he would help us by doing with us the first US EVAR at Montefiore. It worked out perfectly.

I have talked a lot about that seminal moment of Parodi's appearance in New York, the obstacles we faced to get him there, and how important it was to vascular surgery. Thereafter, our meeting always served as a central gathering place for the endovascular pioneers—masters like Juan Parodi, Claudio Schonholz, Julio Palmaz, Thomas Fogarty, Klaus Mathias, Peter Bell, Michael Dake,

Christoph Nienaber, Max Amor, Claude Miahle, Tim Chuter, James May, Geoff White, Barry Katzen, and many others including more recently younger superstars in the field.

Another memorable VEITHsymposium moment: At the 2003 meeting, Bob Dole, who had been a presidential candidate seven years earlier, came as the luncheon speaker and gave an excellent address. He centered his talk on his experience receiving an aortic endovascular graft—an EVAR (at the Cleveland Clinic) for an aortic aneurysm. His appearance was a big success and helped our meeting gain some public recognition. The Dole address also demonstrated the remarkably good relationship our meeting had with industry, and how industry helped physicians improve the care of vascular patients.

Years later, we put on a wonderful event to celebrate the twenty-fifth anniversary of Parodi's first EVAR and the twenty-third Anniversary of the first US EVAR at Montefiore. It was an epic event, extraordinarily well received by all in attendance. The originally cool reception that EVAR had received from the vascular surgery community was blown away by the warm receptions these anniversaries received from all in attendance. The paradigm shift in treatment, which no one had anticipated, had clearly occurred.

At the time of this writing, I can hardly believe that our symposium has completed its *forty-eighth* year and is planning for its forty-ninth meeting. Producing the event is an enormous amount of work, a full-time job requiring twelve months to get the meeting fully ready. Always at my side is our bright and multitalented managing director, Jackie Simpson, a tireless administrator who runs many of the logistics, keeping us on track and faithful to our objectives.

Once I construct the content of the program, Jackie places it on the web, sends out invitations, and works with me to make it perfect. She's also involved in some of the legal and contractual issues, as well as overseeing expenses and accounting. Additionally, she deals skillfully with all our faculty and industry supporters. It's quite a job.

While the symposium has been primarily led by me and Jackie over the last three decades, there are many other key contributors involved who have played a major role in making our enterprise so successful.

Among those whose stellar work should be recognized are Julie Harris, who has been with me since 1974! She is amazingly competent and smart, fully understanding the political and non-clinical issues involved in my professional activities. Julie takes care of our meeting's registration and a number of other administrative details. She has been an essential contributor to the meeting.

I should note that Julie and Jackie were originally my superstar executive assistants at Montefiore, both also acting as my eyes and ears to avoid the many political traps that were set for me.

I should also mention a stellar nurse practitioner, Jamie Goldsmith-McKay, who was for many years my partner in resolving difficult patient and practice issues arising in the office. I would say that Jamie, Julie, and Jackie were my most trusted colleagues (as well as close friends) in all aspects of our professional life.

When you add up Jackie, Julie, Jamie, and my clear-thinking and creative wife Carol—you get a brilliantly dynamic and loyal team, acting with impeccable judgment and incredible efficiency.

Any success I have enjoyed was only possible because of them. In addition, in the last several years, Dr. Enrico Ascher, Dr. Ken Ouriel and Dr. Sean Lyden, the symposium co-chairmen, have been extraordinarily valuable contributors who have participated in the meeting's planning and success in many crucial ways.[24] More recently, Dr. Mark Adelman, a senior vascular surgeon, has joined our organization as an important contributor in several areas. He has been particularly helpful with issues related to program preparation and distribution of the online version of our program, a version we consider a virtual textbook.

I sometimes compare these individuals to a team which manages to win the Super Bowl or the World Series. After a successful clinical year or a winning symposium, I would often say, "Well, we did well this year, but we have to improve and innovate even more so we can win again next year!"

At this point, I remain the senior member of the team with an eye toward our long-range future. In fact, I spend 90 percent of my work time on the symposium, putting my heart and soul into it, working harder than ever to make it survive and thrive. With this in mind, while I am not planning to retire or step down, we've put into place a succession plan that will allow for the continuity and growth of the meeting long after my tenure. It is our hope and plan that the VEITHsymposium will continue on in perpetuity, remaining a

---

24 Since 2006, our meeting has been owned and operated by the VEITHsymposium LLC. Our meeting is sponsored and CME accredited by the Cleveland Clinic, which is, per Accreditation Council for Continuing Medical Education (ACCME) guidelines, responsible for assuring that we follow ACCME guidelines and handling all financial matters related to the meeting (i.e., accounts payable and receivables and providing CME certificates to attendees).

premier vascular meeting worldwide. The staffing may change, but hopefully the quality never will.

To that end, Enrico Ascher has become increasingly familiar with how the meeting is put together and run. He has initiated and directed innovative new adjuncts to the meeting such as our webinars, the Associate Faculty programs and the VEITHsymposium Bulletin. In addition, he has a wealth of creative ideas for how the symposium can maintain its leadership position as an important force in continuing vascular education. So it is most appropriate that Dr. Ascher has been designated as the chairman to succeed me.

As I look back on nearly a half century of our symposiums, I can see how they have been instrumental in keeping our field infused with energy, information, and innovation. Vascular surgeons and specialists must never remain static or myopic in their practice, but must always look to the future to find better ways of caring for vascular patients. This is why a meeting such as ours has been essential for education and progress in the vascular field. Hopefully it will remain that way long into the future and constitute a major part of my legacy.

So far VEITHsymposium has been the fulfillment of a dream, with all vascular specialists under one tent, learning from one another. My wish is that this dream continues and expands to the betterment of all. That is, all physicians involved in vascular disease management, and especially to the people who matter most: the vascular patients we serve and care for.

CHAPTER EIGHT

MENTORSHIP: THE LASTING LEGACY

T he art of medicine cannot be taught from a book.

Yes, academic excellence and steadfast diligence are mandatory during the grueling eight years of college and medical school. It's a grind of morning-to-evening classes, lab work, and in-depth study—training that lays out all the basic groundwork.

But it's hardly enough.

What follows medical school boot camp are the internships and residencies, on-the-job training that is crucially impactful. There is no substitute for it. And when it comes to the field of vascular disease, with all its permutations, complexities, and complications, it's virtually impossible to simulate training or treatment techniques through a book or a session on Zoom.

Only when you have eye-to-eye clinical training under an experienced physician or surgeon can a medical student grow into a competent healer.

As I learned in my early days as a surgical resident, the trained attending surgeon or senior resident guides you through every procedure and operation, correcting your mistakes and fine tuning your techniques, hopefully doing so with patience and respect.

TEACHER/MENTOR TRUTHS

For decades, as a professor of surgery at Albert Einstein College of Medicine and chief of the vascular surgical service at Montefiore, I took the job of teacher/mentor most seriously, and strove for perfection in this role. I should emphasize that teaching is important, but it is only a small part of being a mentor. A good mentor also has to be unselfish and patient. As a teacher/mentor, I would demand the highest standard from my fellows and residents. As I have mentioned, I was even known to some as the White Shark—intimidating and constructively critical to a fault.

While teaching styles *do* differ, the motive beneath them does not. All teaching physicians want their students to grow and to excel and to fulfill their greatest potential. But surgical specialties are not easy disciplines to conquer. As I know too well, when a young surgeon jumps into the deep end of treating patients, it's sink-or-swim. And your teacher/mentor is your life raft, someone who demonstrates how to expertly diagnose and treat patients, how to perform open surgical operations, endovascular treatments, and postprocedural care—how to decide in every detail what to do and not to do.

That's why mentorship is such a crucial component in the training of every young surgeon. A surgical mentor should be a role model, a highly seasoned guide with a proven record of success who can advise on every aspect of medical life—in the emergency room, in the operating room, in the angiography suite, in the examining room, in research, and in the hospital.

A good mentor should be like a great conductor or coach,

leading his players to achieve the optimum result. In the operating room, for example, the mentor is managing every aspect of highly complex surgical operations, showing his or her mentees how to execute each step of the procedure optimally.

In research, a mentor should demonstrate how to organize and conduct clinical studies and how to gather and analyze data. When it comes to documenting the research results, a mentor should guide mentees in their research and in interpreting and documenting their findings. This includes oral presentations, the writing of abstracts and articles, and dealing in a positive way, at times, with rejection. Additionally, trainees have to be guided in conceptualizing new studies and follow-ups to previous ones.

On the behavioral side, a mentor should also be a public-relations guide—someone who demonstrates to mentees how to navigate relationships with patients, staff, other doctors, and hospital administrators.

Importantly, a mentor must also become an ethical compass, teaching young mentees how to analyze the practice of clinical medicine and related scientific research. Students learn that medical ethics are based on a set of values. They must know them backward and forward so that they can resolve any confusion or conflict.

When you put it all together, being a medical or surgical mentor is a weighty responsibility. And it takes a special talent and unselfishness to step into that role. When you take young doctors under your wing, they look at you almost like you are the Tom Brady of your field—someone at the peak of your abilities, an "athlete" doing your best work and then asking *them* to replicate it or improve on it. It can be intimidating.

Beyond being a source of technical skill, a surgical mentor is also an emotional support system. This is paramount. After all, the long hours and the life-and-death nature of surgical care puts a special kind of pressure on the psyche of every doctor.

We often witness tragic surgical outcomes, and endure conditions that are beyond our control. In those pressured moments during often endlessly long days, the mentor is a young doctor's most trusted guide and role model, a shoulder to lean on, someone he or she can observe and turn to for advice and perspective.

In moments of doubt or turmoil, a mentor boosts confidence and teaches survival and leadership skills—demonstrating the value of hard work, discipline, unselfishness, and being tough when you need to be. In short, that mentor expresses the spirit of generosity, conveying that the mentee's welfare is paramount.

To sum it up, a great surgical mentor . . .

- IS CONCERNED AND EMPATHETIC, able to express a genuine sense of caring, listening to both professional and personal problems;
- LEADS BY EXAMPLE, as a positive role model, allowing a young physician to model their ethics, values and standards;
- SHARES PROCESSES—knowledge of medical culture, procedures, office protocols, and overall philosophy;
- IS NON-COMPETITIVE AND CELEBRATES THE MENTEE'S ACHIEVEMENTS, and is never threatened by a mentee's success;
- MOTIVATES to establish goals and help mentees reach their potential;
- KNOWS WHEN TO WAIT before giving advice;
- IS A GOOD LISTENER AND ASKS THE RIGHT QUESTIONS, reading body language and state of mind—you listen to subordinates, following their good ideas and rejecting the bad ones;

- IS OPEN-MINDED, and controls their own emotions;
- IS FORTHCOMING about their own mistakes;
- EXPOSES A MENTEE TO OUTSIDE ACTIVITIES like continuing medical education, classes or projects, books, events, people, etc., to hone a mentee's skills and foster networking;
- IS ENCOURAGING, and enhances confidence and self-esteem;
- PROVIDES GUIDANCE UNCONDITIONALLY, with no expectation of payback;
- IS AVAILABLE AND PATIENT;
- IS SENSITIVE, because tact and diplomacy are crucial in addressing a young doctor's fears and weaknesses;
- IS RESPECTFUL, knowing when not to push too hard is critical;
- IS FLEXIBLE, because you can't control anyone or anything and must shift and adapt with varied circumstances;
- IS SUPPORTIVE—he or she should express pride for what the mentee has accomplished, and in some cases, helps the mentee through board exams, giving them mock oral exams, etc.; and
- IS LOYAL, supportive of the mentee, maintaining confidences, and creating a team mentality.

MY MENTORS
AND SOME MORE GENERALITIES

It is absolutely true that not all surgeons or interventionalists are created equal. Some are poor and only marginally competent. Some are adequate and helpful while others are truly superlative, like one early superstar vascular surgeon, the renowned Dr. E. Stanley Crawford, who I was fortunate to get to know well. I regarded him as an admired friend and the best vascular surgeon in the world.

To put his contribution into perspective, Dr. Crawford, more than anyone in the world, added immeasurably to understanding the complex diseases of the aorta. In fact, surgeons throughout the United States and abroad (including me) traveled to observe his highly refined surgical techniques and skilled manual dexterity, which earned him his reputation as a master surgeon.

Thousands of patients are living happy, productive lives as a result of his contributions, both directly, as their personal surgeon, and indirectly, through his teachings to other vascular surgeons.

I'd often visit him in Houston to watch him in action. Then I'd come back to Montefiore and I'd try to repeat what I had seen. But he was unique; I certainly couldn't replicate some of the things he could do.

Yet slowly, over a period of years, I was able to duplicate some of his skills and accomplish what needed to be done. (Later in life, I really got to know Dr. Crawford well when we served together on the Joint Council of the SVS, with me as treasurer and him as vice president, and later as president.)

Another one of my key mentors was Dr. Francis Moore, a giant of twentieth-century surgery as detailed in Chapter 1. Moore made profound contributions to the care of critically ill surgical patients and the development of organ transplantation programs. In addition to his brilliant and creative research, Dr. Moore was a technically gifted surgeon who performed his operations rapidly and bloodlessly, even in the most challenging of cases.

Dr. Moore mentored me throughout my residency in the care of all sorts of surgical patients. But we really became close during my chief residency, when he taught me administrative and managerial skills. On a personal level, he also taught me how to handle untoward events calmly and effectively in and out of the operating room.

As the Moseley Professor of Surgery at Harvard Medical School and the surgeon in chief at Peter Bent Brigham Hospital in Boston, Moore was also one of the preeminent surgeons in the world. To sum it up, he was good at everything in and out of medicine—a true leader and a star. He was also a most charismatic speaker.

Another of my very important mentors was Dr. Dwight Harken, an internationally acclaimed cardiac surgeon and professor at Harvard Medical School. Dr. Harken had been one of the first to remove foreign bodies from the hearts of soldiers during the Second World War. He also developed a closed-heart technique for surgically treating mitral stenosis resulting from rheumatic fever. This mitral stenosis was a leading cause of cardiac disability at the time. In his technique, he placed a finger into the left atrium of the heart and manually separated the fused cusps of the stenotic mitral valve.

At first the majority of patients died. However, as the method was refined, the mortality rate dropped and the procedure became safe and effective. Harken's concept was adopted worldwide and improved the chance of survival for these patients.

I emulated Dr. Harken in my attitude about training and rewarding my junior colleagues and trainees—giving them maximal responsibility, if they could carry it. As I learned from Harken, a good mentor allows residents to do everything that they *can* do.

Under his brilliant tutelage, I must have done a hundred cardiac operations, most involving severe mitral stenosis. He would guide me during critical parts of the operation—and allow me to take care of patients perioperatively too, which was a real confidence builder.

His service became a model for my own vascular surgical service, based on the way he standardized his operating room protocols, always giving residents the autonomy to do everything they possibly could during operations.

Of course, he was always overseeing every one of our moves and finishing aspects when necessary. In everything he did, he conveyed his trust to the residents and instilled loyalty to him. (As an aside, because Dr. Harken had red hair, we, as his greatest fans, used to tease that we should all dye our hair red, or wear red toupees! We had a lot of fun joking around, even while working very hard.)

There were two other physicians who had a huge impact on me, encouraging me toward vascular surgery. First there was Dr. Chilton Crane, whose wartime service was rewarded with two Bronze Stars, after which he returned to Harvard and the Peter Bent Brigham Hospital. He was the quintessence of the careful, competent surgeon and professor of surgery, dealing largely with disorders of the blood vessels—even though vascular surgery was not then even a subspecialty.

Dr. Crane's principal satisfactions were the welfare of his patients and assisting residents with their early learning process in the operating room. The many generations of surgeons that came under his sway held him in their highest esteem as a teacher of the precise manual skills and detailed anatomic rearrangements that characterize surgery of the blood vessels. I based my operating room behavior on his calm, cool demeanor even when encountering complications and adverse circumstances.

I also met Dr. Richard Warren, who was an equally talented, remarkably skilled surgeon, an inspiring teacher, an author of a leading textbook of surgery, and a devoted member of the Harvard Medical School faculty for fifty years. He was also a most affable, easily approachable person to his trainees. Like Dr. Crane, Dr. Warren had served during the war and became expert at caring for the solders with whom he served. His primary interest also lay in the surgery of blood vessels—especially arteries. During his career, Dr. Warren fostered three major revolutions in vascular surgery: angiography, anticoagulation using heparin, and arterial prosthetic grafting. Disturbed by the careless methods then in use for restoring ambulation by amputees, Dr. Warren also promoted the establishment of a national program for amputee rehabilitation.

As competent as Dr. Warren was, he was quite volatile in the operating room. Ignoring this as much as possible, I tried to model my surgical behavior and protocols on his techniques, but not his reactivity in the operating room. For the latter, I modeled my behavior after that of Dr. Crane. I tried to be calm under adverse conditions because that kept everyone else calm and resulted in the best outcomes for patients.

Another one of my mentors we met in an earlier chapter was the great Dr. Joseph Murray, a Brigham plastic surgeon who was awarded the Nobel Prize for his work in kidney transplantation. His congenial personality, calm demeanor and technical skills as a transplant surgeon were enviable and I tried to copy them.

Although all the Brigham surgeons were decent human beings, Murray, Crane, and Warren stood out in this regard and always treated me and the other Brigham residents with respect and collegiality.

Likewise, the illustrious Dr. John R. Brooks was another attending surgeon who set a great example as a generous mentor. He was a giant of a man, close to six and a half feet tall, who exuded good cheer, often punctuated with a marvelous reverberating laugh.

Having been trained under Francis Moore, Brooks once

allowed me to be first author on an important paper in the *New England Journal of Medicine* (*NEJM*) on thyroid cancer. Dr. Moore had wanted Brooks to be first author because it was an important Brigham paper. I pleaded with Brooks because I had done 95 percent of the work on the paper and written it in its entirety. Brooks went to Moore on my behalf. In the end, I was allowed to be the lead author on this widely quoted and important article.

In addition to interactions with these superstar attending surgeons, it was often the highly experienced senior house staff who acted as junior mentors on the job. They consistently made wise suggestions for solving difficult clinical and technical problems. I would listen carefully and almost always followed their suggestions—usually with good results. When I became an attending surgeon, I tried to copy the willingness of these attending and senior resident surgeons to delegate responsibility. So, when my trainees made innovative suggestions—I listened. Most of the time their ideas worked too.

However, at Montefiore on one occasion, a senior vascular fellow suggested a maneuver to get out of a difficult situation. I followed his suggestion and it got me into much worse trouble (serious venous bleeding). I managed to resolve it, but it was daunting. In this case, I never should have listened to him.

Overall, when I got into serious technical trouble in the operating room, I usually called my colleagues for help, and generally we solved the problems together. Likewise, when they got into trouble, they always called on me.

As time passed, there were many instances when I had to protect my junior colleague partners (attending vascular surgeons) as we coped with the inevitable resentments and jealousies that erupt in any institution. For example, we were sometimes sharply criticized by our general surgery superiors. But I always supported my colleagues, knowing well that the general surgery superiors were *not* as skilled as we, their so-called subordinates.

I believe that these frictions between surgeons were a product largely of jealousy. Why? Because our vascular group, which had pioneered techniques I've discussed in previous chapters, was so successful, clinically and academically. During those times of attack, we had to stick together like a band of brothers in a Marine platoon, fighting in a somewhat hostile environment to support one other, which we did—even to a flaw. Sometimes human emotions got the best of even good doctors! Once when one of my junior attending partners and our interventional radiologist colleague were arguing over who would perform a procedure (a vena cava filter insertion) on a patient, I tried to moderate with my administrator witnessing the discussion.

The argument became very heated. The two physicians came to blows after one called the other an insulting epithet. I jumped in between the two combatants. Punches were thrown, but none landed on them or me. One of the fighters tripped and fell. We all went to our neutral corners, and I said, "Gentlemen, this never happened." I said this because knowledge of the incident and the slur would have led to a doctor being fired. It remained hidden, and no dire consequences followed.

MY ROLE AS MENTOR

If all goes according to plan in the mentor-mentee relationship, one day the roles will reverse themselves; a talented mentee will *become* a mentor, someone who will return the favor and pay back the largesse received. That happened to me in 1971, when my role in life suddenly shifted, and I became chief of my own service at age forty. Instead of being subject to the bosses, I now became a boss and recognized that one of my duties was to become a mentor.

For five decades, I have put a huge amount of time and energy into helping young surgeons, giving them all the tools that they need to become the best vascular surgeons possible. It is one of the most gratifying things I've ever done.

My role as a mentor always started with gauging each trainee's skill level, allowing them to perform parts of operations after observing me do them multiple times. Just as Harken had taught me, sometimes I did half of a particular step and the resident or fellow would do the other half. Or I would let them take over entirely, while I watched. Of course, I would always complete a critical part of the operation.

It always gave me an immense amount of satisfaction when a young trainee could master a surgical procedure. And even when they fell short or failed, I reassured them that they could eventually match or surpass my skill level.

Through it all, I considered my mentees true surgical *partners*. We may not have been equal in skill at the start. But their abilities grew exponentially as we became ever closer, comrades in battle against disease.

In countless hours spent together over a period of years, we shared everything—lead authorship of medical journal articles, research development credit, clinical cases, accolades, money (as they became attending surgeon partners), rewards—everything but our wives!

It reminded me a little of my days in the army as the chief of surgery. Then, as now, we all stuck together—working most of the day and half the night in our quest to provide superlative patient care. Through all the hours spent together in the pursuit of this goal, the relationships with fellows, senior residents and junior partners became very close. It was almost like being married to each other. In the high-tension environment of a working hospital, we essentially lived, ate, and did almost everything together. A close relationship and camaraderie were everything. Despite all the pressures in our work environment, I must say that there was always an element of pure *fun* in mentor relationships. Sometimes I would have the trainees over to the house for drinks or get-togethers, but not as often as I would like. There was just too much work to do. But we had some very memorable parties at Christmas and in the summertime, events that were fun and personal. At ceremonies for graduating fellows, we even roasted one another—all in good humor!

Outside the operating room, when it came to research, we brainstormed together non-stop: We would first conceptualize an idea for a clinical research project—something new and different that we were doing successfully for our patients. Then we would work together to complete the data gathering, write an abstract, and sell it as a presentation and a published article. I make it sound kind of matter of fact, but the entire process was enormously time consuming and presented challenges all along the way.

Some of the most meaningful articles our group wrote were total collaborations with mentees. In 1988, the first journal article appeared on my unique method for treating prosthetic arterial graft infections. This article was published in the *Journal of Vascular Surgery* (*JVS*), entitled "A modified classification and approach to the management of infections involving peripheral arterial prosthetic grafts."[25]

---

25   Samson RH, Veith FJ, Janko GS, Gupta SK, and Scher LA, "A modified classification and approach to the management of infections involving peripheral arterial prosthetic grafts," *Journal of Vascular Surgery* 1988: 8(2): 147–153.

But for years prior to this, I had tried to get our findings published in a good journal but was repeatedly rejected. Why? Because my concept of leaving some, all, or a portion of infected arterial grafts in place went against the grain of then-current medical thinking and beliefs. Yet I knew the method worked because I had used it successfully for many years.[26]

In 1985, in preparation for publication, I asked Russell Samson, a trainee and then a junior attending, to collect all of our data and write an article on my iconoclastic way of classifying and treating prosthetic arterial graft infections—a method which achieved wound healing with preservation of arterial flow via part or all of the involved graft in about two-thirds of appropriate cases.

Samson wrote the article, but it was repeatedly rejected by good journals. He then left our institution to go into private practice, and gave up on the article altogether. But I did not give up. Instead, I rewrote the article several times, and, after many revisions, finally got it accepted in the *JVS* in 1988.

At this point, I had to decide who should be its first author. Should it be me (having conceived of the method and worked so hard to get the article finally accepted) or Samson, who had collected the data and written the first version of the paper. It seemed to me best to have Samson be the first author because he had done the work of assembling the data and written the first version. It is gratifying to me as a mentor today that the classification system is

---

26 I had first described it in 1979, in a chapter (Surgery of the Infected Aortic Graft) of a book edited by Mark D. Morasch, William H. Pearce, and James S. T. Yao, *Surgery of the Aorta and Its Body Branches* (Grune and Stratton, page 521). But no one had paid much attention to this chapter, and it was not indexed. So, I wanted it published in a first-line journal.

now known as the Samson classification system of prosthetic arterial graft infections.

Another example was a 1994 article published in the *Annals of Surgery* on managing prosthetic graft infections. Titled "Selective Preservation of Infected Prosthetic Arterial Grafts: Analysis of a 20-year experience with 120 extra-cavitary infected grafts," it detailed our iconoclastic way to preserve all or part of infected prosthetic (cloth) grafts used to conduct large artery blood flow.

Before this work, it was considered mandatory to remove the entire graft involved with an infection. However, I found that this was not always necessary if one removed (debrided) all the infected tissue from around the graft, kept the wound clean and open, and allowed healing to take place. (First author credit on this concept went to Dr. Keith Calligaro, with me listed as second author.) Notably, this work was presented before the American Surgical Association—the most prestigious surgical society in the world. As the lead author and presenter of this important innovative work, this published paper greatly enhanced Dr. Calligaro's academic visibility and stature.

Thus, my method and the related classification system, which are now widely accepted, are largely attributed to Calligaro and Samson. Promoting the career advancement of junior colleagues is what mentors should do. Doing so is usually very positive, although occasionally one has to give up some credit for one's original concepts and contributions. However, it is a small price to pay for the reward it brings. Dr. Calligaro and Dr. Samson have gone on to prominence and renown in vascular surgery. Seeing their rise within our specialty has been for me one of the great rewards of mentorship.

This was also the case with a 1995 article presented at the American Surgical Association and published in the *Annals of Surgery*, entitled "Initial experience with transluminally placed endovascular grafts for the treatment of complex vascular lesions." This work detailed our initial experience with EVGs for the treatment of all sorts of arterial lesions. Much of this work, done in collaboration with Dr. Parodi of Argentina, was the first of its kind in the world. I decided first authorship should go to Michael Marin, at that time a junior but talented colleague who had trained as a fellow with me and then joined our group as an attending vascular surgeon.

As you remember from a previous chapter, together I and Dr. Marin had started our Montefiore endovascular graft program after doing the first EVAR in the US with Dr. Parodi. Largely on the strength of our innovative work with EVGs, Dr. Marin was recruited to New York's prestigious Mount Sinai Medical Center, where he ultimately went on to become chairman of that institution's entire department of surgery.

For sure, Dr. Marin's surgical, research, and administrative talents made him richly deserving of this position; and seeing him attain this level of success was one of my most gratifying rewards of mentorship.

A similar situation occurred with our original articles on very distal bypasses to ankle and foot arteries. I asked Dr. Enrico Ascher to be first author on many of these articles although I had pioneered many of the techniques before he was associated with our group. I felt he deserved this prominent position because he added creative nuances, collected the data, did several of the cases, supervised the artwork, and wrote some of the articles. Dr. Ascher has gone on to leadership positions and greatness in vascular surgery. He has produced groundbreaking innovations of his own in limb salvage surgery and vascular imaging and guidance with duplex ultrasonography, thereby avoiding exposure to radiation. His leadership has been recognized with the presidency of multiple prestigious organizations. These include the Society for Clinical Vascular Surgery, the Eastern Vascular Society, the World Federation of Vascular Societies, and the Society for Vascular Surgery. We remain close friends and colleagues, and he has played a major role in the recent executive direction of the VEITHsymposium. His great success is most gratifying to me. It represents one of the best fruits of mentorship.

During my Montefiore years, in most of our presentations at prestigious societies and their matched articles, I tried to share the spotlight with mentees as much as possible—and much more than did many of my colleagues in similar positions

In fact, as illustrated above, I often made my junior colleagues *first* author on a concept that I originated and developed. Sometimes I took a great deal of heat on new concepts because they were the result of out-of-the-box, against-the-grain thinking—for which I usually was the main recipient of the doubt and skepticism.

Examples other than those already mentioned are our work on a very aggressive approach to salvage threatened limbs, distal origin bypasses, prosthetic lower extremity bypasses including those to lower leg and foot arteries, unusual surgical approaches to lower extremity arteries with scarring or infection, the value of redo and multiple redo procedures for failures, the failing or threatened bypass graft concept and its treatment, the value of extended extra-anatomic bypasses, and all our original work with surgeon-made EVGs. All these procedures were not done in numbers before we did them and all were generally not accepted when we first described them. Although I received the negative reactions and skepticism for introducing these procedures, it was gratifying to see my colleagues ultimately get credit for them—credit which I took pleasure in sharing. However, more commonly after we introduced

a new concept or procedure, those outside our group claimed the credit as the innovators. I guess they forget where they first heard or read about it. Such folks often honestly believe they thought of the new concepts and procedures. Such is human nature.

Often when I gave my mentees first authorship on key articles, it was because they had worked hard on one of our concepts and I felt they deserved the credit. More often, particularly later in my career, it was because I wanted to advance *their* careers.

In the same vein, my general thinking was that it was better to include colleagues as an author than to leave them off a presentation or article. I always felt that sharing rewards was a key aspect of leadership. As it turns out, I believe that sharing the byline was one major reason why so many of my trainees and colleagues went on to have very successful careers, which included top positions at hospitals, in medical schools and in vascular societies.

I also believed it was my role as a mentor to share our interesting and challenging cases, as well as the financial, academic, and research rewards. I felt that such generosity would make me a better leader, keep my colleagues happy and productive, and ultimately enhance the reputation of our service and our institution. I always believed that my performance as a leader would be measured by the success of my mentees and the group I was leading.

Thus, to succeed as a mentor and chief in vascular surgery requires a different mind-set than that needed to succeed as an individual vascular surgeon. The latter can have "me-centered" goals and strivings and justifiably care mainly about his own achievements, rewards and career advancement. However, the former must have "we-centered" goals and strive to advance the career and rewards of those under his or her leadership. Although I know such a policy will work in vascular surgery and lead to the greatest group achievement and rewards, I suspect that these principles will also apply to other medical specialties and all other circumstances where leadership is required. A successful group is like a family. Affection and mutual support continue even when the members leave the group to go to different institutions.

In short, a great mentor or chief must fight for their team members. This requires unselfishness. Everyone must be treated fairly, and the leader must devote time and effort to making that determination accurately. Leaders must put their team members' welfare above their own, and gain rewards in the collective output of the group and the success and reflected glory of the individuals under their direction.

Yet in the US today, it is often only about serving self-interest.

But one must go beyond ego to have the best interests of one's mentees at heart. Mentorship is all about training a colleague to follow in the mentor's footsteps well enough to have the mentee actually *exceed* the mentor's accomplishments.

On that note, no matter how much I might have *given* to mentees, I think I've *gotten* a lot more in return. That's why the mentor-mentee relationship is a two-way street. Yes, I did everything I could to train them and help them in their subsequent career; and in return, they gave back with their accomplishments, skill, and success. (At the end of this chapter, some of the individuals I have mentored share some of their experiences working with me.)

Many of these former trainees, as you have and will read, have gone on to illustrious careers, successfully heading up departments or services and gaining officer positions in prestigious societies. It is for me the ultimate gratification to see them become leaders in our specialty and beyond.

As time passed and I got a little older, some of my mentees wanted my job before I was ready to retire. One of my partners thought I should step down at age fifty. When my ninety-year-old father stopped by our office on his way to his busy law practice in Manhattan by subway, during New York's high-crime years, my partner gave up calling for my early retirement

There are still other advantages to be gained by a mentor who treats his mentees well and unselfishly. Firstly, they represent a lasting legacy. Whereas one surgeon and his accomplishments and innovations are soon forgotten after his passing, a group of younger mentees will keep them alive and pass them on to their trainees and mentees. One's influence can thus be magnified and perpetuated indefinitely—a real and meaningful legacy.

Secondly, one surgeon, no matter how hard a worker, can only accomplish so much. However, a *group* of surgeons working together and with the same goals can accomplish much more and can conquer almost any challenge. That was why I believed it was vital to create such a group—or dynasty—and why it was so important to give full and continuing support to all its members.

On a final note, while mentorship of young doctors was a vital part of my professional life, so also was my surgical practice, research, writing, academic travel, and leadership roles at the hospital and in professional organizations. As a result, I am sorry to say that I sometimes neglected my familial duties back at home. I was often an absentee husband and father.

Beginning in the late 1950s, my wife Mary and I had our four children in quick succession. Throughout this time, I was consumed by work, for which I paid a big price. First in Boston as a resident, later in the army, or back in New York, I left most of the parenting to Mary, who was a smart woman and a very good mother.

We had married in 1955. But because of my commitment to work, the family relationship suffered. Yes, I appreciated the kids when they did well in school or athletics, but unlike some of my friends, I was just not a natural hands-on dad. Mary and I divorced in the seventies. In the past several decades, I have tried hard to be loving and more supportive of my four children and my twelve grandchildren. I am pleased to say that these grandchildren include one lawyer, two vascular surgeons in training, a psychologist, a dietician, a certified public accountant, a real estate agent, two computer science experts, a banking executive, a nurse practitioner, and a pharma executive. I am indeed proud of these children and grandchildren!

Several years after my marriage ended, I met a bright, wonderful lady named Carol LaMantia, a nursing supervisor at Montefiore who worked in the dialysis and transplant unit. We first met when she made an appointment to consult with me about being a kidney donor for her sister. We hit it off right away and married in 1980. Our relationship has been a great blessing and source of happiness in my life.

I've asked a few of my mentees to write their accounts of working with me. This, in my view, details my mentorship better than I could myself.

KEITH CALLIGARO

Chief, Vascular Surgery and Endovascular Therapy,
   Pennsylvania Hospital
Program Director of Vascular Surgery Fellowship,
   Pennsylvania Hospital

FRANK J. VEITH, MD

Clinical Professor of Surgery, University of Pennsylvania
Past President of the Society for Clinical Vascular Surgery
Past President of the Eastern Vascular Society
Treasurer of the Society for Vascular Surgery

In the spring of 1986, I walked into Dr. Veith's office at Montefiore Medical Center to interview for a vascular surgery fellowship position. His administrative assistant led me into his inner sanctum and I gazed around the office, seeing piles of manuscripts and journals and books splayed out on all of his bookcases, chairs, and desk. I wondered how anyone could keep track of this mess! Then I felt a whirlwind of energy as Dr. Veith walked quickly into the office, shook my hand, and sat down.

For the next hour, he fired away questions at me while taking phone calls and yelling commands to his administrative assistant. I was just trying to keep up and occasionally get a word in. He concluded the interview by telling me I was a good guy before calling his physician's assistant to give me a tour of the hospital. I caught my breath and thought, "I never met anyone with as much energy as that guy." And thirty-five years later, Dr. Veith still has more energy than anyone I know.

In addition to his infectious energy, there are other facets of his personality that shaped my career over three decades. Once I was accepted into the program, I spent hours writing and re-writing my first abstract to make it absolutely perfect. I proudly gave Dr. Veith my masterpiece. Then, over the next few minutes my smile disappeared as his pencil darted across the paper crossing out unnecessary verbiage and adding succinct phrasing. He handed me the pencil-covered paper with arrows and slashes, got up, and walked away without a word.

I stared at what he had done to the best abstract ever written, got angry that he destroyed my work, and then slowly realized that in just five minutes he had rendered the "masterpiece" that I had labored over for hours into an immeasurably better abstract. I realized I had a long way to go. Now serving on the editorial board for the *Journal of Vascular Surgery*, I never review or write a manuscript without thinking of his editing acumen. I try my best to emulate his skill, but I know I cannot duplicate it.

In the operating room, Dr. Veith demanded perfection from his vascular fellows. During an anastomosis, if a suture I placed was off by 1 mm, he would *gently* and *kindly* remind me (these adjectives are intended to be sarcastic) that I needed to do better. He insisted on obtaining as perfect an outcome as possible; anything less was unacceptable. To this day I find myself taking my trainees through operative cases as meticulously as he did (although in a slightly gentler, kinder manner).

During my time with him at Montefiore, Dr. Veith's positive attitude regarding patient care and surgical outcomes was contagious. He would make rounds with the vascular team, always making positive remarks in a strong rat-a-tat voice. He'd then leave with a thumbs-up gesture to the patient. To this day I can't stop myself from giving that same thumbs-up gesture to patients when I leave their rooms.

Truly, he is the strongest patient advocate I have ever known. He has always spoken strongly against performing unindicated interventions and reminds all of us to act in the patient's best interest. He often calls interventionalists who do unindicated procedures "criminals."

Dr. Veith has strongly encouraged his trainees to remain academically productive, and he remains as dedicated to teaching trainees and other vascular surgeons today as he was fifty years ago.

Inspired by his VEITHsymposium, I have served as program director of our accredited vascular fellowship for thirty years. I know I would not have become president of the Society for Clinical Vascular Surgery and the Eastern Vascular Society, or treasurer of the Society for Vascular Surgery, without his mentorship and guidance.

Dr. Veith has more passion for vascular surgery than anyone I know. He always instilled this passion into his trainees, as evidenced by the fact that all of his past fellows are out there defending vascular surgery as a specialty and defending patients from non-vascular physicians who pose as vascular specialists.

In summary, Dr. Veith's energy, editing ability, positive attitude, desire for surgical perfection, patient advocacy, academic encouragement, and above all, passion for our specialty, illustrate why Dr. Veith is the quintessential mentor for all vascular surgeons.

MAHMOUD MALAS

Professor and Chief of Vascular Surgery,
   University of California, San Diego

Dr. Veith is a visionary surgeon, an exceptional mentor, and a magnificent human being, someone who has become a guiding light to everyone who worked with him. But due to his innumerable accomplishments, he *can* be intimidating. Yet those who know him intimately understand that he is someone who always stands by his principles and is never afraid to go against the tide (a true visionary in adapting and developing endovascular surgery as an alternative to open procedures).

My first interaction with Dr. Veith came about back when I was doing my general surgery residency at USC and looking for a fellowship position. Back then, the Montefiore fellowship under Dr. Veith was *the* most competitive such fellowship in the world. And though I had a small chance of being accepted for it, I canceled a conflicting interview at the University of Tennessee. Being the rebel that I was, I held the belief that I was equally capable, if not more, than any other candidate applying for the position!

On the day of the interview, in my excitement, I arrived so early that only Dr. Veith was in the office. My excitement was short-lived! As the interview began, what Dr. Veith said practically squashed any hopes I had of landing this job. In his usual challenging demeanor, he began by telling me that there were several hundred applications for this *one* spot in his program, and that he had narrowed the field down to just ten.

"Can you prove to me that you have what it takes and convince me that you are the best among all these candidates?"

I thought to myself, maybe I *had* made a mistake coming for this interview! I could not possibly be the best candidate out of those top ten. But since I believed I had already lost the battle, I decided to enjoy the ride while it lasted. Instead of getting intimidated by his question, I challenged him in return.

"Dr. Veith," I said. "I *also* have had several interviews in the top programs in the country and today *you* should convince *me* why your program should be my number one choice for training!"

This was the first time in our exchange that Dr. Veith actually paid any attention to me. A lot of people in his position would have squashed anyone who dared to challenge them. But Dr. Veith saw my assertiveness as a positive quality and did not take offense to it. After all, he was accustomed to people agreeing with him on *every-thing*, so my bold statement set me apart. In fact, despite my being a barely-out-of-the-operating room surgical resident, saying what I did was one of the main reasons I got hired (even though I had an unfamiliar name and came from an unusual background).

But Dr. Veith was way ahead of his time in terms of inclusion and diversity, so he was not bothered by my name. And he was certainly not afraid to go against the grain, even if it meant hiring someone who clearly did not fit the usual profile of a surgeon during that era. What mattered to him were my credentials and performance, not what was visible on the surface. And this trait remained consistent throughout the fellowship.

The work wasn't easy. He commanded excellence and expected nothing less from his mentees, which is why sometimes they also faced the brunt of his tough love, though I always found him to be extremely respectful. We would often round on the patients together and review their angiograms/imaging. He would always turn to me and ask, "So Mahmoud, what do you think about this angio, what should we do?"

For me, this was mind-boggling. Here was a pioneer in vascular surgery asking his fellow for an opinion on the patient management?! But it was always his habit to make me feel part of the team and that stimulated me to learn more.

The most beautiful thing about Dr. Veith's mentorship is that *it never really stopped*. When I was looking for my first job after the fellowship, he strongly insisted that I take up an academic position rather than going for private practice or other financially superior options. It was because of him that I ended up taking the job at Johns Hopkins, which launched my career in academic vascular surgery. And he was right in his foresight.

During my time at Hopkins, I had incredible opportunities to build the endovascular program from scratch and begin numerous clinical trials. And through it all, I could always count on Dr. Veith to have my back, a unique trait in a field as closely knit yet competitive as vascular surgery.

Even today, I can call him on a Sunday and he will take my call and take time to listen and provide his expert advice on whatever it is that I am struggling with. He extends the same treatment to all his mentees, the kind of mentorship I strive to provide for my trainees.

To sum it up, Dr. Veith is an excellent educator who has played a pivotal role in molding the careers of three generations of vascular surgeons, many of them leaders today. So, through his impact, his influence lives on. I am forever indebted to him for the training that I received because it shaped me into the vascular surgeon that I am today.

PALMA SHAW

Vascular Surgeon, Brigham and Women's Hospital

Assistant Professor of Surgery, Harvard Medical School

Professor of Surgery and Vascular Surgery Program director, Upstate University Medical Center, State University of New York in Syracuse, NY.

Secretary General, World Federation of Vascular Societies

I first met Dr. Frank Veith in 1999 when I asked him for advice about applying for a vascular surgery fellowship position. He reviewed my application and said I would be competitive for his program and inspired me to apply. He wound up offering me a position to work in his lab as a Visiting Scholar/Research Fellow in Vascular Surgery. I was thrilled.

I remember that year well (2000–2001) for so many reasons, viewing it as a turning point in my career. Every Tuesday during office hours, he taught me so much. I always will remember that he said "you had to sit down to properly assess pedal pulses," the beat of the heart as felt through the walls of a peripheral (foot) artery, such as that felt in the radial artery at the wrist. And I still assess patients that way.

When we discussed cases, he always wanted *my* opinion about what to do, always making me feel like a valued member of the team. As for the work ethic, when you work for Dr. Veith, even for *free* as I did that year, you were expected to always be available to him. I had to buy a beeper just for him in case he wanted to reach me.

During our routine research meetings on Tuesday afternoons, he had us present all of our projects and progress for the week. Those meetings went on for hours but I never minded because he worked even *harder*.

With deadlines for abstracts coming up for the annual meeting of the Society for Vascular Surgery, it was crunch time in December. I was home making Christmas Eve dinner and Dr. Veith called me to go over the abstract. I dropped everything to work on it because that is what he expected. I was just happy to be involved with his research.

At the VEITHsymposium meeting that year, he asked me to sit in the front row just in case he needed me to do something to help the meeting run smoothly. I was glued to the chair. And I learned so much from *his* meeting, while every subsequent academic vascular meeting seemed redundant, a carbon copy of what he had already covered.

And most amazing to me, the VEITHsymposium was a parade of the "who's who" in vascular surgery, the giants in our field who I felt honored to meet. Sometimes they would be visiting the lab to collaborate with Dr. Veith. I would never have interacted with them had it not been for him.

Overall, it was a great time of progress for endovascular aortic aneurysm repair devices and research. I learned a great deal of cutting-edge material from him, which helped me significantly during my formal vascular fellowship at Newark Beth Israel Medical Center.

When I was finishing my year with him, he wanted me to stay another year. But I told him that I could not afford to as I was working with no stipend. He laughed, but he was right! I would have loved to continue working with him.

Ever since then, I have attended almost every VEITHsymposium during my career, fortunate to participate in a number of them as a presenter or moderator.

When I changed positions to a new university hospital, I often discussed the challenges I was having in adjusting to a new team. To help me understand why I felt unwelcome, he would tell me that I was the "new Gorilla in the cage," and gave me advice about how to acclimate myself to my new partners, reminding me that these things take time, and that I just had to be strong and persistent.

Finally, one wonderful thing about Dr. Veith is that he likes to have fun! For example, in 2011, at an endovascular conference held in Shanghai, we both attended a reception complete with dancing and costumes. Dr. Veith was the life of the party, dancing on the stage! He was having a great time. Then, again, in 2019 at the VAST3 meeting, he took center stage on the dance floor once again. So as much as he was laser focused on work, he would punctuate our interactions with fun too.

On a final note, as a woman physician in the male-dominated domain of vascular surgery, I have felt challenged at times by my colleagues. His support during difficult times was sometimes the only thing that kept me going. I learned the meaning of resilience from him. And although Dr. Veith was the busiest person I know he was always sincerely interested and gave me great advice. Nobody supported me more. Honestly, he has been like a father to me. So, I will always be grateful for his teaching, mentorship, and support.

EVAN LIPSITZ, MD,

MBA Chief, Division of Vascular and Endovascular Surgery
Professor of Cardiothoracic and Vascular Surgery
  Department of Cardiothoracic and Vascular Surgery
  Montefiore Medical Center and the Albert Einstein College
  of Medicine
Past President of the Eastern Vascular Society

I was exceptionally fortunate to train with Dr. Frank Veith at Montefiore. At our first interview, I remember him telling me that it was a revolutionary time in our field, with the ongoing use of the surgeon-made Montefiore endovascular graft system; the first wave of industry-sponsored clinical trials for endovascular aneurysm repair; and the ever-present aggressive approach to limb salvage.

As I soon discovered, Dr. Veith was known for being outspoken. But his other qualities often went underappreciated. For example, he is a staunch advocate for conservative therapies when he believes there is no significant benefit to intervention. I will never forget his tag line that, "All interventions are finite and imperfect." And he practices what he preaches, providing appropriate care with a long-range view in the interest of the patient.

He is also a systematic thinker and able to present diagnostic and therapeutic options in a compelling way that makes perfect sense. Additionally, he is great writer. (As my father told me, good writing is *rewriting*.) I can tell you that our final abstract submissions bore only a slight resemblance to their original iterations! Dr. Veith was a perfectionist and would require that we rework the material. And all that reworking frequently went well into the eleventh hour. In his view, it could always be better.

In the course of research, he asked great questions of himself and of others. I discovered that he had an insatiable curiosity for all things technical—stents, grafts, computers, the new fluoroscope, etc. That curiosity carried over in a very positive way to all of his trainees. While working with us, he also demonstrated persistence in the acquisition of knowledge and skills.

I remember sitting in the audience during Dr. Veith's landmark SVS presidential address and thinking that my fellowship was going to be an exciting and interesting time, which of course, it was. Dr. Veith innovated with foresight, pushed the specialty along, and took an interest in our field in a way that positively impacted all vascular surgeons.

Yet there was a lighter side to all of this too. Despite Dr. Veith's stature and the specialty's respect for him, he was a very good sport, evidenced by his good humor during a good-natured roast of him that took place at the Houston Aortic Symposium in 2013.

All in all, despite his judiciously critical evaluation of our performance, Dr. Veith always displayed introspection and a desire for feedback, particularly related to technical matters. Early in my fellowship, for example, I was doing a difficult bypass with him and he was encouraging me to "foil." (This means placing one's forceps on the outside of the artery wall on either side of the suture needle to support it while suturing a very diseased artery.) He seemed frustrated that I did not seem to know what he meant.

He kept repeating, "Foil, don't you know what foiling is?" Then, after a pause, he quietly said, "Well, I guess I made it up," and on the case went.

On a different occasion he was helping another surgeon do a complicated operation while I was the fellow. His dissections were always meticulous, and the case was proceeding rapidly. Dr. Veith was openly (if not rhetorically) asking whether the other surgeon was too fast or whether he was too slow. He was fascinated with all things relating to President Clinton and how he could "get away with it."

Finally, Dr. Veith's ongoing impact on all of us is perhaps best represented in a quick anecdote. Several of us were together at the hospital when suddenly we got paged. Dr. Veith sighed and said, "It doesn't matter how old you are, seeing that number still makes your heart sink." We all could relate, and just laughed.

NEAL CAYNE
Professor and Director of Endovascular Surgery
NYU Langone Medical Center

When I first began as an intern on the vascular surgery service, I heard the name Veith multiple times a day, but never actually met him. (At that time, he was recovering from a medical procedure.) But the way his dominating and powerful manner was spoken about, it was as if an empire was missing its king. I was quite intrigued.

In my second year, I finally met him. I remember walking into a big office. He was a very direct and articulate man. He perfunctorily asked me a few questions about my training, shook my hand firmly, and told me that he looked forward to me returning to the vascular service.

Our next meeting wasn't until my third year of training, at which point I attended Dr. Veith's infamous Tuesday morning teaching conference. I was forewarned by my senior residents to read the pertinent literature *prior* to attending conference. Sure enough, he called on me and I was ready with the correct answer, inspired to be perfect, both clinically and academically.

In the operating room, he demanded perfection, from the planning of the procedure, exposure, and execution. Every move, every stitch had to be thrown exactly right. If not done perfectly, in Dr. Veith's words, "It just won't work!" and had to be redone.

During one procedure, I worked so diligently to make him proud, but every stitch I threw was not thrown correctly. I was not able to follow his suture the way that he liked. I remember him yelling at me to "FOIL." I had no idea what that meant, having never heard the term in the operating room.

Finally he screamed, "Don't you know how to foil???"

To which my response was, "No, Sir."

He then calmly said, "OK, then let me show you . . . this is a single foil, this is a double foil. . . ." (It turns out to be a fencing term.)

One day after that procedure, I received a call from one of the vascular attendings telling me that Dr. Veith was very impressed with my performance on the service and wanted me to consider a career in vascular surgery. I was in shock that he thought highly of me. But I went ahead and did choose vascular surgery as a specialty.

I stayed at Montefiore with Dr. Veith to do a vascular fellowship, and am extremely grateful for his teaching and mentorship. He taught me how to write papers and how to be meticulous in everything I did, most importantly as a safe surgeon. He also emphasized the importance of being a good diagnostician as well as a good vascular surgeon. I can recall him asking a patient with an inflamed toe the last time that he had his uric acid checked—looking for gout, not a vascular surgery problem.

A good portion of what Dr. Veith taught me, I still practice today and try to pass on to my trainees. As he always said, you have to be not only a great surgeon, but a *safe* one. For example, Dr. Veith once got into a jam disrupting a large lumbar artery while circumferentially dissecting an aorta. He developed a safer way to clamp it. His surgical technique and surgical theory stay with me today on each and every case I perform.

As the years passed, my relationship with Dr. Veith matured from one of being fearful of him (or fearful of not being good enough to impress him) to one of great friendship. I can now share things with him about my life and family outside of vascular surgery that he can appreciate. During training, nothing other than vascular surgery seemed important to him. He will always be a true mentor to me both clinically and academically. I will always cherish what he taught me, the surgeon that he guided me to become, and now the more personal relationship that we have come to develop. He is a true mentor, and I hope that I can come close to emulating him with my trainees.

CARLOS H. TIMARAN

Chief, Endovascular Surgery
Professor of Surgery
Sam H. Phillips Jr. MD Distinguished Chair in Surgery
    University of Texas Southwestern Medical Center

I first had the opportunity to attend the VEITHsymposium in 2000, the conference held at the magnificent Waldorf Astoria in New York City. At the time, I was a third-year general surgery resident at the University of Tennessee Medical Center at Knoxville, fascinated by the meticulous surgical techniques and the artful skills required for vascular exposures and repairs. At the event, I was surrounded by the best vascular surgeons in the world and even had the chance to ask Dr. Veith a question, which he answered in his typical polite, precise manner. Interacting even briefly with the master of masters was enough for me.

A year later I actually interviewed for a fellowship at Montefiore under Dr. Veith. As I observed him on rounds, I could see how he approached his patients in a thorough, compassionate, and understanding manner, so clearly communicating the details of the patient's condition and options for treatment. He did *not* influence their choice of treatment, but rather provided them with all the information necessary to make informed decisions.

I was also impressed by his thorough and detailed physical exam, everything about it so efficient and meticulous. While checking for pulses, for example, he insisted that the patient had to lie completely supine, with the arms on the side, the head and neck relaxed and in a neutral position. He demonstrated to his trainees how the pulse in the feet could disappear when the patients raised their heads. To this date I continue to implement this technique.

At the end of the interview day, and while Dr. Veith and I were walking out of the hospital, he kindly told me that his executive secretary Jackie said good things about me.

"She likes you," he said, "and that's a good thing."

I would soon observe that one key to his success was implementing the team approach, which allows him to delegate and maximize productivity. As I grew to know him better, I observed the unbiased character of a man who recognized the courage, hard work, and persistence of his team. Never was there any bias based on gender, race, ethnicity, nationality, or place of origin.

During the second year of fellowship, I noted that Dr. Veith always took on the most challenging vascular cases with optimism and pragmatism. One of the most striking features of observing any of Dr. Veith's surgical procedures was his utter confidence in performing optimally. Early failures, takebacks to the operating room, or immediate revisions were extremely rare, as he insisted on the utmost meticulous execution of the procedures with extreme attention to detail. That discipline has proven key to the success of any of the complex procedures I perform today, and one of the features I strive to relay to my own trainees.

One day during a complex case, Dr. Veith was holding a guide-wire for me. I asked him to release it to advance it into a target vessel. Because of my strong accent, sometimes I would raise my voice to speak firmly. At one point, he approached me and whispered in my ear: "The next time you yell at me, please consider that I may certainly put you out of business . . ." I understood the importance of respectful and effective communication in the operating room. I felt embarrassed and apologized. Years later I have meditated on his words. How true they were.

During this period, I saw that Dr. Veith could get key expert advice on the phone, whether in government, medicine, or the sciences. His influence was unparalleled. Toward the end of my fellowship, when I was looking for a job, I mentioned two important institutions that were of interest to me. He asked the nurse in the operating room to call Jackie and get the chiefs of those services on the phone. Within minutes, Dr. Veith had them both on the phone, telling them how strongly he supported my application and his belief that I would one day be a "superstar." Whether or not *that* was true, I was so grateful to have his unconditional support.

Ever since I finished my fellowship and started my academic career at the University of Texas, Southwestern Medical Center in Dallas, Dr. Veith and I have been in continuous communication. Like any great mentor, he frequently checks in with me about my clinical cases and congratulates me on my successes. I can only hope to live up to the impeccable standards that he has set as a surgeon, researcher, and mentor—always demonstrating courage, dedication, and persistence, even in the face of adversity. Having Dr. Veith as my mentor is one of the most distinct privileges of my career, while having his friendship and support are priceless.

EPILOGUE

LOOKING FORWARD

Now in my senior years, I look back on the entire story of my life and feel a deep sense of thankfulness.

I once read that gratitude is the prayer of the enlightened. I really believe that. Count your blessings, not your sorrows. You have to be grateful for whatever has been given to you. And first and foremost is the gift of health.

I'm sometimes surprised by how young I feel, still vitally energetic and driven to serve in any way I can, most notably now in the production of the VEITHsymposium.

Do I miss doing surgery? Some days I do, as there is nothing more gratifying than performing an operation that works, one that saves a patient's life or limb. I look back on thousands of such procedures that changed the course of lives forever, and I am glad I had the privilege of being able to help.

Beyond the day-to-day surgical routine, I am still engrossed in all aspects of my field. I confer constantly with my mentees and other vascular surgeons about their patients and advances in vascular procedures; I still devour medical journals, follow research developments, all of it feeding the variety of our symposium topics, all of them centered on the desire to heal the human body.

If only I could have healed some of the human psyches I've

encountered! As you've read, my push to advance cutting-edge techniques in limb salvage, lung transplantation, and endovascular procedures were often met with surprising skepticism and even hostility. Who would ever think that a hospital staff, other surgeons, and vascular specialists could be as competitive as football teams? Probably more so. In my experience, people were often vying for power spots, public attention, grant money, and better offices, ruthless in their pursuit of self-gain, attention, and prestige. Even worse, revolutionary vascular techniques were often denigrated or ignored, the status quo being like a bottle to a baby. The Medical Mafia fiercely held a tight grip on to its old rituals, even preventing vascular surgery from becoming an independent specialty, even though it was and is a no-brainer.

Am I bitter about it? I never have been. And I don't have time to be. Yes, I've been deeply frustrated that others have resisted the advances I advocated that were ultimately proven correct. And sadly, I've also known many doctors and medical administrators who demonstrated self-interest and poor judgment—who resented progress and defied indisputable new research and clinical findings. They were trapped in the loop of the past, resisting progress at almost any cost, afflicted with the diseases of jealousy, greed, and resentment. This only shows how flawed human nature can be.

Even when the *New York Times*, the *Wall Street Journal,* and other publications clearly supported our mission to make vascular surgery an independent specialty, the medical establishment continued to dig their heels in, defying the initiative at any cost. As I see it, their negativity was usually self-serving. We see similar behavior in our politics, in our legal system, and in the medical community too.

But as a counterbalance to all that, I am blessed to have known hundreds of fine physicians, researchers, and hospital staff members who have demonstrated the highest level of integrity. They work tirelessly in operating rooms, angiography suites and in research laboratories, only interested in finding better treatments and perfecting surgical and interventional techniques. Instead of being driven by ambition or their egos, they lead with compassion and a genuine desire to heal. And yet every day, those people face those who would thwart their efforts for various reasons.

The ultimate *goal,* of course, is improving the health of patients. They are the ones we should care about most. They are the ones who should come first. And so it remains to this day.

Despite my chronological age, I still feel passionate about serving the public health effort—society's needs. Accidental or not, my destiny, it seems, was to become not only a doctor but a researcher, an innovator, and a leader who always went against the grain, advocating for what I felt was right. I will never stop. And I hope that the doctors who I have worked with and who support me will carry on their work in years to come, guided by our main priority, which is to improve the health of our vascular patients.

ACKNOWLEDGMENTS

As you've seen, this book traces the history of seven decades of medical study, research, pioneering surgeries, and the battle against the Medical Mafia. Putting all this into a book was a formidable task, and I have many thanks to give.

Most importantly, I thank my wife of forty-two years, Carol, who is a loving partner, a friend, and an insightful advisor. Throughout my career and the evolution of this book project, she has provided help, support, and wisdom.

I am also profoundly loving and grateful to my children and grandchildren, who had to tolerate my excessive commitment to work. I am very proud of them and their accomplishments. Their achievements and successes please me greatly.

A special debt of gratitude goes to my longtime public relations manager and advisor, Pauline Mayer. Over the last twenty-two years, Pauline has done an outstanding job promoting the VEITHsymposium while tending to a plethora of other public relations projects. Pauline helped prepare the initial research materials for this book. She thereafter creatively managed the marketing and public relations in conjunction with the publisher.

As far as the actual writing of this book is concerned, I want to thank my brilliant collaborator—bestselling author Glenn Plaskin, who created a fluent narrative that captured my voice and experiences. His diligence, insight, and commitment to the project made him altogether indispensable. In our many months working together, we developed a true friendship.

I want to thank the team at Amplify Publishing, including CEO Naren Aryal and production editor Brandon Coward, who meticulously edited, designed, guided, and produced the book in your hand. I am also indebted to the expert editing of Zachary Gresham, who skillfully melded multiple drafts together with insight and efficiency. I also thank the Amplify public relations team, headed by Kristin Perry and Sky Wilson.

In addition, I give heartfelt thanks to my home team members who have supported and guided me for decades:

First, there is Jacqueline M. Simpson, managing director of the VEITHsymposium. Undertaking a herculean task with multiple talents, she handles her many duties brilliantly each year with organizational skill and finesse that are second to none. She has been a trusted confidant and friend for years in her many executive capacities.

Next, I thank Julie Harris, also a trusted confidant and friend, who is the director of VEITHsymposium registration. For forty-two years, Julie has served in stellar fashion as my extraordinarily skillful executive assistant. In the course of writing this book, she supplied valuable research and writings.

I want to also acknowledge my longtime nurse practitioner, Jamie McKay, who was a remarkably capable associate and a staunch patient advocate with skills in the management of vascular disease superior to most of my physician colleagues. She was always a trusted advisor and friend. For good reason, she was loved by patients and respected by our trainees.

The initiatives chronicled in this book and the colleagues who participated in them could not have succeeded without the profound loyalty, skills, and commitment of the young women who served as our executive secretaries and assistants: Nancy Yates and June Gitstein in the early years, followed by Julie Harris, Jamie McKay, and Jackie Simpson. They were collectively the glue that held our group together and kept us working in both the academic and clinical realms. They finalized our articles and grants, managed our schedules, helped us take care of our patients, and alerted us to impending challenges from without. Without their contributions there would be no team and no successes. I and my colleagues are forever indebted to these remarkable women.

I must also thank the extraordinary Enrico Ascher, MD, who is a VEITHsymposium co-chairman—a physician and surgeon whose skills and creativity in vascular surgery exceed mine. He richly deserves all the leadership positions he has been awarded in our specialty. I greatly appreciate and value his friendship and support.

Thanks to Kenneth Ouriel, MD, who is another VEITHsymposium co-chairman. He is a preeminent vascular surgeon who has achieved noteworthy leadership, academic and business success in our field.

My appreciation also goes to Sean Lyden, another leading vascular surgeon and the other co-chairman of our VEITHsymposium. I am most grateful to Sean for his supportive leadership and for helping our meeting maintain the extremely positive relationship it has enjoyed with the Cleveland Clinic.

Deep gratitude also goes to my vascular surgery partners over the years. We truly were a band of brothers and sisters.

I also thank the mentee-colleagues mentioned in Chapter 8, who kindly offered their memories about working with me. I do believe the greatest thing a physician or surgeon can do is to train another, and I was privileged to be their guide. My legacy rests with all my colleagues and with them.

APPENDIX

SINGLE-LUNG TRANSPLANTATION IN EMPHYSEMA

Originally printed in *The Lancet*, May 1972.

F. J. Veith

S. K. Koerner

L. A. Attai

P. Bardfeld

S. J. Boley

A. Bloomberg

M. Everhard

J. Anderson

B. Pollara

R. Steckler

H. Nagashima

S. Siegelman

P. Lalezari

M. L. Gliedman

SUMMARY

A patient with severe bilateral emphysema has survived more than 3½ months after receiving a single-lung allograft. At least seven presumed episodes of rejection were identified and reversed by massive pulsed intravenous doses of methyl prednisolone. When allograft rejection was controlled, no serious or progressive ventilation-perfusion imbalances occurred and the allograft provided the majority of effective ventilation and pulmonary blood-flow, with consequent improvement in the patient's respiratory status.

INTRODUCTION

Allotransplantation of a single lung in patients with emphysema has uniformly been fatal. Most of the patients have died with pulmonary insufficiency associated with a marked ventilation-perfusion (V/Q) imbalance characterised by overperfusion and underventilation of the transplant. This has generally been attributed to the presence of a transplanted lung in parallel with an emphysematous lung which has an abnormally high static compliance, expiratory airway resistance, and vascular resistance.[1–3] In this setting, the bulk of the pulmonary blood-flow has been distributed to the compressed transplant, while the majority of ventilation has occurred in the overexpanded emphysematous lung.[2] Since the perivascular mononuclear-cell infiltrates typical of allograft rejection have not been present in many of these patients, this V/Q imbalance was thought to be due to the physiological setting and not to rejection.[1–3] For this reason, a bilateral procedure has been considered essential if lung transplantation is to be successful in the treatment of emphysema.

Unmodified lung-allograft rejection is associated with alveolar exudates and mononuclear-cell infiltrates concentrated in and around blood-vessels.[4,5] The former constitute the principal alveolar manifestation of rejection and produce decreased transplant ventilation; the latter represent a vascular manifestation of rejection and are associated with impaired transplant perfusion.[5] In unmodified lung-allograft rejection, the alveolar and vascular manifestations progress simultaneously,[5] and transplant ventilation and perfusion are both impaired. Recently, we have presented evidence in animals and man that immunosuppression may attenuate the vascular manifestations of lung-allograft rejection to a greater extent than the alveolar manifestations.[5–7] Thus, lung-allograft rejection under immunosuppression could produce impaired ventilation without decreasing allograft blood-flow. On this basis, we have suggested that rejection contributed more than was previously thought to the V/Q imbalance and fatal respiratory insufficiency in emphysematous recipients of single-lung transplants.[7] If this is true and if rejection could be controlled, a single lung allograft in an emphysematous patient might not be associated with serious V/Q imbalance.

We describe here the results of allotransplantation of the right lung in a 53-year-old man with severe bilateral emphysema.

CASE-REPORT

For three years before operation, the patient had required ventilatory assistance with a volume-cycled respirator via a cuffed tracheostomy tube. Despite inspiratory pressures of more than 50 cm. of water and an inspired oxygen concentration (F.I. O_2) of 40%, the patient's arterial oxygen tension was as low as 46 mm. Hg and his arterial carbon-dioxide tension ranged from 60 to 100 mm. Hg.

Since the fourth week after transplantation, the patient has been able to breathe comfortably without ventilatory assistance and without a tracheostomy. While breathing ambient air (F.I. O_2 21%) spontaneously, he has been able intermittently to maintain an arterial carbon-dioxide tension of 39–44 mm. Hg and an arterial oxygen tension of 66–71 mm. Hg for the past fifteen weeks. A perfusion scan (see accompanying figure, top line) was performed twenty-four days after operation by injecting 2 mC of ^{99m}Tc-labelled human serum-albumin in the form of micro-spheres (15–30 m) into a peripheral vein. This showed that the bulk of the pulmonary blood-flow was distributed to the transplanted right lung. A ventilation scan (figure, centre line), performed by having the patient breathe into a closed spirometer system containing 10 mC of xenon-133, showed that the transplanted right lung was ventilated more rapidly and more evenly than the emphysematous left lung. A washout scan (figure, bottom line) was performed by allowing the patient to breathe xenon-free air after the xenon-133 content within the patient's lungs and the spirometer had come into equilibrium. This showed that the xenon-133 was removed more rapidly from the transplanted lung than from the emphysematous lung.

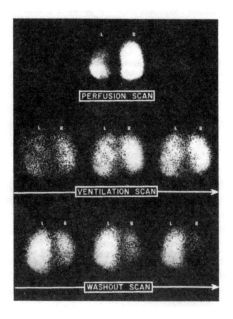

Radioisotope Scans Twenty-Four Days after Right-Lung Allotransplantation. The top line shows the results of the perfusion scan; the centre line shows the sequential results of the ventilation scan at thirty-second intervals; and the bottom line shows the sequential results of the washout scan at thirty-second intervals.

Despite immunosuppression with azathioprine (2–3 mg. per kg. per day), prednisone (1 mg. per kg. per day), and rabbit anti-thymocyte globulin or horse antilymphoblast globulin (13–30 mg. per kg. per day for thirty-one days), the patient has had at least seven apparent episodes of rejection of his allografted lung. These have been characterised by dyspnœa, an increase in body-temperature (102–104°F), the appearance of an infiltrate on chest X-rays, a decrease in the arterial oxygen tension, and a need for increased inspired oxygen concentrations in the absence of any significant change in the number or character of organisms present on culture or smear of the tracheal secretions. All the manifestations in each of these presumed rejection episodes have been completely reversed by supplementing the patient's immunosuppressive therapy with 1 g. doses of methyl prednisolone given at twelve-hourly intervals for two to four days. Antibiotic drugs have not been required during any of these apparent rejection episodes.

COMMENT

These findings show that a single-lung allograft can be of therapeutic value in emphysematous patients. They also indicate that serious V/Q imbalances do not occur merely because of the presence of a transplanted lung in parallel with an emphysematous lung. Thus, the experience with this patient militates against the necessity for bilateral transplantation in emphysema and substantiates the premise that rejection was a more important cause of failure in emphysematous recipients of single-lung allografts than has heretofore been recognised.

REFERENCES

1. Wildevuur CRH, Benfield JR, "A review of 23 human lung transplantations by 20 surgeons," *Ann. Thorac. Surg.* 1970; 9: 489–513.

2. Stevens PM, Johnson PC, Bell RL, Beall AC, Jenkins DE, "Regional ventilation and perfusion after lung transplantation in patients with emphysema," *New Engl. J. Med.* 1970; 282: 245–9.

3. Bates DV, "The Other Lung," *ibid* 277–79.

4. Barnes BA, Flax MH, Barr G, "Experimental pulmonary homografts in the dog," *Transplantation* 1963; 1: 351–64.

5. Veith FJ, Sinha SBP., Blümcke S, Dougherty JC, Becker NH, Siegelman SS, Hagstrom JWC, "Nature and evolution of lung allograft rejection with and without immunosuppression," *J. Thorac. Cardiovasc. Surg.* 1972; 63: 509–20.

6. Siegelman SS, Dougherty JC, Hagstrom JWC, Sinha SBP., Veith FJ, "Radiological dissociation of alveolar and vascular phases of rejection in allografted lungs," *Ann. Thorac. Surg.* 1971; 12: 127.

7. Veith FJ, Hagstrom JWC, "Alveolar manifestations of rejection: an important cause of the poor results with human lung transplantation," *Ann. Surg.* 1972; 175: 336–48.

EASTERN VASCULAR SOCIETY PRESIDENTIAL ADDRESS

TRANSLUMINALLY PLACED ENDOVASCULAR STENTED GRAFTS AND THEIR IMPACT ON VASCULAR SURGERY

Frank J. Veith, MD, from the Division of Vascular Surgery, Department of Surgery, Montefiore Medical Center & Albert Einstein College of Medicine, New York, N.Y. Presented at the Eighth Annual Meeting of the Eastern Vascular Society, Montréal, Québec, Canada, May 12–15, 1994.

surgery (n.,): The branch of medicine that deals with the diagnosis and treatment of injury, deformity and disease by manual and instrumental means.

radiology (n.,): The use of ionizing radiation for medical diagnosis, especially the use of x-rays in medical radiography and fluoroscopy.

war (n.,): A condition of active antagonism or contention; a concerted effort to put an end to something considered injurious.

cooperation (n.,): Joint effort or operation; the association of a number of people in an enterprise for mutual benefits.

compromise (n.,): A settlement in which each side gives up some demands or makes concessions.

Sources: Webster's and New Heritage Dictionaries.

It has been a pleasure and a great honor for me to serve as president of the Eastern Vascular Society for the past year. It is my firm belief that the Eastern Vascular Society will become increasingly important to vascular surgeons in the Northeast, and I will take a few minutes from my main topic to tell you why.

Vascular Surgery is being buffeted by the winds of change. Indeed vascular surgery as we have known it is under pressure from a number of directions. First is the declared intent of other specialists in medicine, cardiology, and radiology to take over the care of patients with vascular disease.[1–5] Unfortunately this intent is partly fueled by the desire of some of these other specialists to use their newly found catheter-based techniques more widely. This is particularly troublesome when these techniques are used to treat vascular lesions simply because they exist, without much consideration for their benign natural history or the long-term safety and efficacy of the treatment. Obviously this approach by these interventional "cardiovascular specialists" can be both expensive and harmful and not in the interests of some patients. Second are the efforts of our federal government to tame the health care costs "monster." Medicare reimbursements for vascular operations have already decreased. Further cuts along with incentives *not* to treat are on the horizon as is a broad financial attack on the concept of specialty care per se.

Where does the Eastern Vascular Society fit into all this? Although originally conceived as a scientific society to further the dissemination of knowledge, I believe that the Eastern and other major regional vascular societies must play increasing roles in vascular surgery's efforts to deal constructively with these forces and pressure having an impact on us. The Eastern Vascular Society should become an organization that represents the interests of vascular surgeons and their patients in interactions with the public, with other specialties, and with government, particularly at the state level. To this end we have formed a committee chaired by John Ricotta to deal with these governmental and public relations issues. Hopefully we will all support this committee and the Eastern Vascular Society as a means for dealing with these negative forces better. If we do and some of our efforts succeed, the Eastern Vascular Society may become far more important to all of us than its founders ever thought.

You will note that I have *not* called upon the Eastern Vascular Society to help vascular surgeons adapt in an organizational or political way to the impact of new technologies. This it can only do by disseminating scientific information and related concepts as it has done from its inception. The remainder of my remarks today will hopefully do just that, namely provide information and derivative concepts that help vascular surgeons adapt better to the impact of a new technology, endovascular stented grafts.

Transluminally placed endovascular stented grafts or TPEGs is a terminology that refers to a concept, a technology, and a group of devices. The concept is to insert via a remote access site, far from the vascular lesion requiring treatment, a new prosthetic vascular conduit, to guide it within blood vessels into position, and to anchor it there with suitable fixation elements in a way that the vascular disease is repaired in a less invasive fashion than would characterize a standard operative approach. TPEGs can be used in the arterial or venous systems, and they can employ autogenous, biological, or prosthetic conduits. Today I will restrict my discussion to prosthetic TPEGs that are used in the arterial tree.

The TPEG concept was first expressed in 1969 by Charles Dotter, the pioneer of fluoroscopically controlled angioplasty and other catheter-directed techniques.[6] Throughout the 1980s several investigators explored the use of TPEGs to treat experimental aneurysms in animals.[7–10] In 1985 Nicholas Volodos, a Russian surgeon, first used a TPEG device with a self-expanding stent to treat iliac arteriosclerotic occlusive disease.[11] However, his work, published only in Russian, received scant attention until Juan Parodi, an Argentinean surgeon, performed the first TPEG repair of an aortic aneurysm in a patient at high risk in September 1990. This original successful case along with five others was reported in 1991 by Parodi and his two associates, Julio Palmaz, a radiologist and developer of a balloon expandable metal stent, and Hector Barone, an Argentinean developer-manufacturer of vascular grafts and other related devices.[12]

The clinical TPEG program at Montefiore and Einstein began in November 1992 under the leadership of Michael Marin and Frank Veith with the collaboration of several vascular surgeons (Thomas Panetta, William Suggs, Ross Lyon, Luis Sanchez, Kurt Wengerter, Steven Rivers, and Michael Schwartz) and two interventional radiologists (Jacob Cynamon and Curtis Bakal) and support from Parodi's Argentinean group (Juan Parodi, Claudio Schonholz, and Hector Barone).

To date our group has inserted 62 TPEGs in 43 patients with a variety of aneurysmal, occlusive, and traumatic lesions at different sites within the arterial tree (Table I).[13–20] All the patients with aneurysmal and occlusive disease and most of the patients with traumatic lesions had some major medical comorbidity or a surgical problem (scarring, infection, or other organ disease) that precluded standard surgical or interventional treatment. Many were not candidates for general or regional anesthesia. All but one patient had some open vascular surgical component to their procedure.

Nine of these 43 patients (Table I) had abdominal aortic or aortoiliac aneurysms that were considered categorically inoperable after careful cardiopulmonary and surgical evaluation. Two patients had iliac artery aneurysms. One patient had a popliteal aneurysm. Nine patients had traumatic false aneurysms without or with an arteriovenous fistula. Eighteen patients received unilateral or bilateral ($n = 3$) TPEGs for aortoiliac and femoropopliteal occlusive disease that was causing limb-threatening ischemia. Twenty-one of these TPEGs were placed in the aorto-iliac-common femoral segment, although eight of these extended to the superficial femoral or popliteal arteries. Four additional patients received isolated femoropopliteal TPEGs for limb-threatening ischemia. Our femoropopliteal experience was paralleled by the work of Cragg and Dake,[21] although their TPEGs were inserted percutaneously largely in patients with intermittent claudication and less extensive disease.

Our techniques for performing these TPEG procedures and the early results extending now to 18 months have been or will be reported in detail elsewhere.[13–20] Even though many of our early cases had end-stage disease with multiple previous therapeutic failures, our results to date have been encouraging. Although three of the 43 patients have died of their comorbid cardiopulmonary disease several months after their TPEG procedure, all 12 of the patients with trauma and non-aortic aneurysm have effective, functioning TPEGs from 1 to 18 months (mean 10 months) after their procedure. Five of the nine aortic or aortoiliac aneurysm TPEG procedures were and continue to be successful, but two of the patients died after their procedure, one of multiorgan failure and one from microembolization. Of the 21 aortofemoral or iliofemoral grafts, 19 remain patent. One patient died of unrelated causes with a patent graft, one graft failed, and five grafts required minor reinterventions yielding a 1-year life table secondary patency rate of 94%.

However, this experience is still too scant to make any recommendations about widespread use of these endovascular methods or to suggest that our indications be broadened to include any but these otherwise untreatable patients. Moreover our overall experience to date allows us to emphasize a few generalities that anyone wishing to enter this alluring new field should consider. Almost all these TPEG procedures were complex and difficult to perform. All required and taxed the combined skills of those who regard themselves as expert in the techniques of open vascular surgery and the catheter-guidewire-imaging skills of interventional radiology. Successful attainment of a satisfactory endpoint frequently necessitated a major vascular surgical or catheter-guidewire "rescue" component to the procedure. All these procedures were performed with an anesthesiologist in attendance and full invasive pressure monitoring in an operating room equipped with a moveable radiolucent operating table and a digital fluoroscope. In several instances this venue and staffing were critical to achieving a successful outcome, because some of the procedures proved to be long, complicated, and associated with major blood loss. Although it is possible that these problems will be obviated by improvements in our relatively primitive devices and technical refinements that come with experience, this has yet to be proven.

Despite these reservations this field of TPEG devices remains one of great interest and indeed agitation and apprehension to vascular surgeons, and it is appropriate to ask "why" and then go on to examine the possible impact of this interesting, still unproven new technology on our field of vascular surgery.

Why are we all so interested in and agitated by TPEGs when we were not as disturbed by balloon angioplasty or even the premature hype about endovascular lasers? Simply stated, balloon angioplasty was applicable to only a small percentage of our surgical cases,[22,23] and lasers never worked very well. However, TPEGs are a potentially better method to treat a major fraction of our surgical cases, and *TPEGs may work*. The recent report of Parodi[24] supports this possibility. So does our work that I have just summarized.[13–20] So also does the report of Moore and Vescara[25] on the preliminary experience with the Endovascular Technologies aneurysm device. TPEGs are less invasive to insert. They are therefore concordant with a major current trend in all of medicine and are inherently attractive to both patients and physicians. If TPEGs do work as well as standard procedures or even nearly as well, they will replace standard vascular grafts. Moreover these TPEG devices offer the possibilities of lower mortality rates, fewer complications, shorter hospital stays, and consequent cost reductions, all of which have great appeal to government and third-party payers. Of course all these potential advantages of TPEGs have to be proven by appropriate comparative performance clinical trials. To this end guidelines for carrying out such trials as part of a systematic and responsible development program for these TPEG devices have been written by the Endovascular Committee of our two major National Vascular Societies.[26] This committee, working with the National Institutes of Health, is also establishing a National Registry to document accurately how well these TPEGs work.

LESION	NO. OF PATIENTS	NO. OF GRAFTS
Abdominal aortic or aortoiliac aneurysm	9	18
Iliac aneurysm	2	2
Popliteal aneurysm	1	1
Traumatic false aneurysm	7	8
Arteriovenous fistula	2	2
OCCLUSIVE DISEASE		
Aorto-iliac-femoral	18	24
(3 Bilateral) (8 to superficial femoral or popliteal artery)		
Femoropopliteal	4	7
TOTAL	**43**	**62**

Table I. Montefiore/Einstein experience with transluminally placed endovascular stented grafts[13-20]

But what if these devices do work and compare favorably with our standard grafts? The percentage of vascular grafts that will be replaced by TPEGs remains to be determined and will be influenced by a number of variables including technologic developments. However, I doubt that TPEGs will be another laser fiasco and that the percentage will be insignificant. My present best guess is that 35% to 70% of current vascular prosthetic grafts could be replaced by TPEGs. That potential and the fact that insertion of these devices requires catheter-guidewire-imaging skills, which we generally do not have, in addition to our vascular surgical skills explains why vascular surgeons are so interested in and yet agitated by TPEGs.

These devices could make vascular surgeons as we currently know them largely obsolete.

How then will vascular surgeons cope with the introduction of TPEGs, and what will the impact of effective TPEGs be on our specialty? Several possible courses of action have been suggested. One approach taken by some is to adopt an attitude of skepticism and denial. "These new devices won't work because no endovascular interventional technique has been any good and none will be. Therefore let's ignore TPEGs as we did lasers, leave them to others to fiddle with, keep doing what we have always done, and not be concerned." This ostrich approach is dangerous and wrongheaded. Interventional procedures can be effective. Balloon angioplasty and stents clearly work in appropriate circumstances. The early experience already cited suggests that TPEGs will work. Moreover the ability to line a thrombogenic arterial lumen traumatized by a balloon and stents with the less thrombogenic, friendlier flow surface of a prosthetic graft increases the possibility of success. If vascular surgeons adopt the ostrich approach and TPEGs do work, they are likely to be excluded from a leadership role in the use of these devices. At best they will be reduced to dealing with complications and providing access to the arterial tree or anastomoses when the profile of the device and other exigencies require open arterial surgical procedure. At worst, except as a clean-up crew to deal with failures that cannot be corrected with an endovascular procedure, vascular surgeons will be excluded entirely as technologic improvements make most TPEGs suitable for percutaneous use. Thus this ostrich approach should be shunned by vascular surgeons.

A second almost as dangerous approach that could have the same outcome is to wait and see how well TPEGs do work and only get into the fray when they are proven effective in a significant fraction of patients undergoing vascular surgical procedures. This approach is founded on two premises. The first is that other interventional specialists[27] are not really interested in inserting TPEG devices in patients with vascular disease without our direct participation. The second is that vascular surgeons have a God-given right by virtue of our knowledge of vascular disease processes and pathology, prosthetic grafts, and how to deal with complications to control these devices, if they do work. These two premises are not true. These other interventional specialists sincerely believe that their facility with catheter-guidewire-imaging techniques qualify them better to insert TPEGs than do our vascular surgical skills and knowledge of vascular disease. This is particularly so if the devices can be made with a small enough diameter or "profile" for percutaneous insertion, as has already been possible.[13,21]

Of course experience to date has shown and most clear thinkers

27　Interventional specialists include interventional radiologists, some cardiologists, and a few vascular physicians who feel qualified to perform procedures in the peripheral arteries. In general cardiologists are trained to deal with the heart and its arterial bed, and some of them (interventional cardiologists) have catheter- guidewire-imaging skills. Although such individuals might be welcome additions to those who treat peripheral arterial disease, they must demonstrate that they have the credentials, experience, and skills not just to treat lesions but to treat patients with these lesions. This requires that they have the training and experience equivalent to that of an interventional radiologist, a vascular physician, or a vascular surgeon and that that training be not only in the performance of angiograms and interventional procedures, as is currently the case, but also in the surgical and conservative noninterventional treatment of patients with vascular diseases.[23] In all subsequent discussions peripheral trained interventional cardiologists and vascular physicians will be included in the group described as interventional specialists or "interventional radiologists."

realize that optimal TPEG effectiveness can be achieved when the devices are used and inserted by those with expertise in vascular surgical and interventional skills. Such combined skills can be provided by teams comprised of vascular surgeons and interventional radiologists. Such teams, largely under the leadership of vascular surgeons, have been responsible for most of the successful TPEG developmental efforts to date. Thus a third approach to TPEGs for vascular surgeons to take is to work with such a combined multi-specialty group that manages all patients with vascular disease in a collaborative fashion. In current practice, with few exceptions, vascular surgeons are responsible for patient care decisions, and most multidisciplinary collaborative groups are presently led by vascular surgeons.

However, we must be concerned over the stated goal of some interventional specialists to change current practice and assume major responsibility for all care of patients with vascular disease.[1–5] Of course the achievement of that goal mandates that the interventional specialist having this major care responsibility would have all the skills, knowledge, and judgment currently possessed by most vascular surgeons. This is not presently the case with most interventional specialists who are largely trained in and oriented toward treating lesions and not patients. This is exemplified by the unfortunately common current practice of subjecting patients with minimal calf claudication to percutaneous balloon angioplasty and even placement of multiple stents. Better knowledge of the benign nature of this symptom would obviate unnecessary treatment in many patients. It is also true that financial considerations have been a powerful incentive for all specialists to treat these patients with minimal symptoms. Moreover financial considerations may work against collaborative team approaches to TPEG placement, because third-party payments may not be adequate for multispecialty participation. Creative solutions to this problem need to be developed.

A fourth and in my opinion the optimal approach to the TPEG problem for vascular surgeons is for them to become sufficiently competent in catheter-guidewire-imaging-stent technique to allow them to perform the entire procedure without interventional radiology support, unless they encounter an unusual problem. This arrangement would be a role reversal for most vascular surgeons and interventional radiologists with regard to current balloon angioplasty and stent placement. It also creates a number of subsidiary problems for most of us. Obtaining appropriate training in these basic endovascular techniques is a fundamental requirement for vascular surgeons and trainees. This will not be easy. However, adequate numbers of vascular surgeons possess these skills to make such training feasible with appropriate organization and an effective administrative structure. Alternatively, many of us have adequate, mutually beneficial relationships with other specialty colleagues so that adequate training could be obtained for us to perform TPEG procedures as part of a healthy collaborative relationship. This does not imply that vascular surgeons should become interventional radiologists or attempt to replace them. It simply means that as vascular surgeons develop improved TPEG techniques for managing vascular lesions, they must also develop sufficient proficiency with catheter-guidewire-imaging-stent methods so that they will be able to use the TPEGs that may replace standard arterial repairs and bypasses.

This issue introduces the sensitive and critically important topic of how the relationship should evolve between two previously distinct specialties as a new technology that truly overlaps both is introduced. TPEGs are such a new technology. Both vascular surgeons and interventional radiologists have legitimate desires and justification to feel that they should control this potentially important new development. Accordingly conflict can result. Such conflict has already occurred, and many believe furious turf battles or *war* is inevitable. However, such a war will be costly and will result in casualties at both the physician level and more importantly at the patient level. If possible, such wars should be avoided. Accordingly I would like to suggest a radical solution based on mutual understanding, *cooperation*, and *compromise*. If it works, all, including patients, will benefit.

First we must examine the fears and concerns of the vascular surgeons and the interventional radiologists. Both are afraid that they will be displaced by the other group, and the fears are legitimate. If vascular surgeons develop catheter-guidewire-imaging-stent skills, some interventional radiologists fear they will become unnecessary and redundant. Vascular surgeons can do most arteriograms and balloon angioplasties, and they can place stents. On the other hand if interventional radiologists can insert TPEGs, and TPEGs work, a major portion of vascular surgery will become obsolete, and some vascular surgeons fear they will become unnecessary and redundant. These fears of both groups are fueled by extremists in both specialties who openly suggest taking over each others' fields. Indeed the outcome of the resulting war will only be determined after it is over—and there will be casualties.

The crucial step in avoiding this conflict is for both groups to retreat from these extremist views, remove the fear factor, and reassure each other by word and deed that mutual destruction is not a goal. Interventional radiologists must be reassured that vascular surgeons do not intend to take over diagnostic angiography, balloon angioplasty, and stent placement as they currently exist. Vascular surgeons must be assured that they will be able to perform TPEG insertions as they replace open vascular operative procedures. Helping us obtain sufficient endovascular training to do this would be a beginning. This and our helping interventional specialists to learn the value and role of other treatments for vascular disease might launch true collaboration where none existed.

However, this will not be enough. Our two specialties have to become unified or confederated at the highest levels and be willing to represent each other's interests in the most basic and critical ways. This will require creation of a Combined Executive Committee of the Joint Council of the Society for Vascular Surgery and the North American Chapter of the International Society for Cardiovascular Surgery and the Society for Cardiovascular and Interventional Radiology. The seed for such a cooperative venture between the two specialties exists in the combined group that participated in the writing of the guideline document for development of TPEGs.[26] However, the proposed new Combined Executive Committee will have to deal with such thorny issues as defining acceptable practice guidelines across the specialties, training each other's members and trainees in areas in which they are weak, and limiting the numbers of trainees so that excessive numbers of specialists are not produced in both fields.

The long-term goal of this collaborative leadership function would be to produce adequate numbers of optimally trained specialists so that our nation's needs for treating vascular disease could be appropriately met. This would work best if vascular surgeons and interventional radiologists of the future worked in combined services or departments of vascular disease treatment led by either a distinguished vascular surgeon or radiologist. These departments would be administratively and financially separate from both surgery and radiology. Members of these departments would distribute their responsibilities for patient care and procedures in an equitable way that was determined within the service or the department in the same fashion that such matters are administered within a surgery or radiology service, department, or group at present. Financial rewards and other forms of compensation would be determined in the same way.

This radical solution will not happen easily. Resistance will come from a number of quarters, and it will take time. However, this solution is intrinsically right. It will reduce costs and provide optimal patient care and treatment by avoiding the splintering of care, financially motivated procedures, and choice of procedure based on an individual physician's training or skills or what resources he or she controls. It will facilitate the evaluation of different treatments. And most importantly it will obviate the need for painful costly wars, the worst possible impact the introduction of TPEGs could have for all of us and our patients.

REFERENCES

1. DeMaria, AN, "Peripheral vascular disease and the cardiovascular specialist," *J Am Coll Cardiol* 1988; 12: 869–70.

2. Kinnison ML, White RI, Auster M, et al, "Inpatient admissions for interventional radiology: philosophy of patient management," *Radiology* 1985; 154: 349–51.

3. Katzen BT, van Breda A, "Developing an interventional radiology practice," *Semin Intervent Radiol* 1988; 5: 99–102.

4. Kerlan RK, Marone T, Ring EJ, "The clinical role of the interventional radiologist," *Semin Intervent Radiol* 1988; 5: 103–4.

5. Cook JP, Dzau VJ, "The time has come for vascular medicine," *Ann Int Med* 1990; 112: 138–9.

6. Dotter CT. "Transluminally-placed coilspring endarterial tube grafts: long-term patency in canine popliteal artery," *Invest*

Radiol 1969; 4: 329–32.

7. Balko A, Piaseck GS, Shah DM, Carney WI, Hopkins RW, Jackson BT. "Transfemoral placement of intraluminal poly-urethane prosthesis for abdominal aortic aneurysm," *J Surg Res* 1986; 40: 305–9.

8. Mirich D, Wright KC, Wallace S, et al. "Percutaneously placed endovascular grafts for aortic aneurysms: feasibility study," *Radiology* 1989; 170: 1033–7.

9. Laborde JC, Parodi JC, Clem MF, et al, "Intraluminal bypass of abdominal aortic aneurysm: feasibility study," *Radiology* 1992; 184: 185–90.

10. Chuter TAM, Green RM, Ouriel K, Fiore W, DeWeese JA, "Transfemoral endovascular aortic graft placement," *J Vasc Surg* 1993; 18: 185–97.

11. Volodos NL, Shekhanin VE, Karpovich IP, Troyan VI, Guriev YA, "Self-fixing synthetic prosthesis for endoprosthetics of the vessels," *Vestn Khir* (Russia) 1986; 137: 123–5.

12. Parodi JC, Palmaz JC, Barone HD, "Transfemoral intraluminal graft implantation for abdominal aortic aneurysms," *Ann Vasc Surg* 1991; 5: 491–9.

13. Marin ML, Veith FJ, Panetta TF, Cynamon J, Barone HD, Schonholz C, Parodi JC, "Percutaneous transfemoral stented graft repair of a traumatic femoral arteriovenous fistula," *J Vasc Surg* 1993; 18: 298–301.

14. Marin ML, Veith FJ, Panetta TF, et al, "Transfemoral endolu-minal stented graft repair of popliteal artery aneurysm," *J Vasc Surg* 1994; 19: 754–7.

15. Marin ML, Veith FJ, Panetta TF, et al, "Transfemoral stented graft treatment of occlusive arterial disease for limb salvage: a preliminary report [Abstract]," Circulation 1993;

88[suppl]: I-11.

16. Marin ML, Veith FJ, Panetta TF, et al, "Transluminally placed endovascular stented graft repair for arterial trauma," *J Vasc Surg* 1994; 20: 466-73.

17. Marin ML, Veith FJ, Cynamon J, et al, "Transfemoral endovascular stented graft treatment of aortoiliac and femoropopliteal occlusive disease for limb salvage," *Am J Surg* 1994; 168: 156-62.

18. Marin ML, Veith FJ, "Endoluminal stented graft aortobifemoral reconstruction," In: Roger M. Greenhalgh, ed. *Vascular and Endovascular Surgical Techniques, an Atlas*. 3rd ed. London: WB Saunders Company, 1994: 100-4.

19. Marin ML, Veith FJ, Cynamon J, et al, "Transfemoral endoluminal repair of a penetrating vascular injury," *J Vasc Interv Radiol* (in press).

20. Marin ML, Veith FJ, "Transfemoral retrograde stent graft repair of abdominal aortic aneurysms: the Parodi Procedure," *N Engl J Med* (in press).

21. Cragg AH, Dake MD," Percutaneous femoropopliteal graft placement," *Radiology* 1993; 187: 643-8.

22. Veith FJ, Gupta SK, Wengerter KR, et al, "Changing arteriosclerotic disease patterns and management strategies in lower-limb-threatening ischemia," *Ann Surg* 1990; 212: 402-14.

23. Veith FJ, Gupta SK, Wengerter KR, Rivers SP, Bakal CW, "Impact of nonoperative therapy on the clinical management of peripheral arterial disease," Circulation 1991; 83[suppl I]: I-137-42.

24. Parodi JC, "Endovascular repair of abdominal aortic aneurysms," *Adv Vasc Surg* 1993; 1: 85-106.

25. Moore WS, Vescara CL, "Repair of abdominal aortic aneu-

rysm by transfemoral endovascular graft placement," *Ann Surg* (in press).

26. Endovascular Stented Graft Committee, "Guidelines for development and use of transluminally placed endovascular prosthetic (stented) grafts in the arterial system," *J Vasc Surg* (in press).

Reprinted from the Journal of Vascular Surgery, *December 1994, Volume 20, Number 6, Frank J. Veith, "Presidential address: Transluminally placed endovascular stented grafts and their impact on vascular surgery," pgs. 855–860, Copyright 1994, with permission from the Society for Vascular Surgery and International Society for Cardiovascular Surgery, North American Chapter, and Elsevier.*

SOCIETY FOR VASCULAR SURGERY PRESIDENTIAL ADDRESS

CHARLES DARWIN AND VASCULAR SURGERY

Frank J. Veith, MD, from the Division of Vascular Surgery, Department of Surgery, Montefiore Medical Center & Albert Einstein College of Medicine, New York, N.Y. Presented at the Fiftieth Annual Meeting of the Society for Vascular Surgery, Chicago, Illinois, June 11–12, 1996.

Selection as President of The Society for Vascular Surgery is for me a singular honor, especially because it comes on the 50th Anniversary of this esteemed Society. However, this is a time of enormous upheaval in American medicine, and holding this office has also forced me to focus on the future of Vascular Surgery and how well it will survive these turbulent times. The resulting concern I have for the future of our specialty has prompted me to select Charles Darwin as the topic of my Presidential Address. It is certainly reasonable to wonder what possible relevance Darwin, the famous English naturalist and the father of the theory of evolution, could have to Vascular Surgery. In fact, the theory and principles of Darwin are important to our specialty, and I will explain why.

THE LIFE AND ACCOMPLISHMENTS OF CHARLES DARWIN

Charles Darwin was born in 1808 to a wealthy medical family in Shrewsbury, England. His father, a fashionable physician, entered his young son in Edinburgh Medical School. However, young Charles fled in horror at the sight of his first operation. Because the choice of alternative careers was limited and his aptitude for the classics minimal, his father enrolled Charles in Christs' College at Cambridge University with the intent that he become a clergyman. At Cambridge, Darwin obtained the rudiments of a scientific education and was able to pursue his boyhood interest in the natural history of plants, birds, and insects. Indeed, until the defining event in Darwin's life, it appeared that he was destined to become yet another botanizing Victorian clergyman. That seminal event was his appointment as Naturalist on the naval ship, *H.M.S. Beagle*, which had been commissioned to make a surveying voyage of the unexplored nether regions of South America, including Patagonia and Tierra del Fuego. This 40,000 mile, 5-year voyage included many adventure-filled inland expeditions that gave Darwin a view of the natural world from the Brazilian jungle to the peaks of the Andes. His observations led him to speculate about the relationship between extinct and contemporary species and to question the then-current view that animal and plant species, having been created by God in His infinite wisdom, are permanently fixed and immutable. Concepts born in Darwin's mind on the voyage of the *Beagle*, together with supporting evidence gathered on that trip, ultimately led to his definitive formulation of the theory of evolution in *The Origin of Species By Means of Natural Selection*, published 23 years after the voyage.[1] Darwin was not one to rush prematurely into print and had spent the two decades between the formulation of his theory and its announcement in wrestling with potential objections and collecting supportive facts. This caution was based on Darwin's recognition that his theory would contradict religious thinking and would therefore elicit a storm of hostility and opposition. As Mark Twain would subsequently say: "Let a man proclaim a new principle and public sentiment will surely be on the other side." This statement certainly applied to Darwin's theory in his era. It is often applicable today, and it may apply to parts of this Presidential Address.

The theory of biologic evolution was not new. By Darwin's own count, evolutionary ideas had been put forth by more than 30 predecessors going back to the ancient Greeks. Others, including Diderot, Lamarck, and Darwin's own grandfather, had previously expressed evolutionary concepts only to have them greeted by theologic indignation and discredited in favor of divine creation of fixed species. Darwin's unique accomplishment was to accumulate a massive body of exemplary evidence, bolstered by the newly emerging scientific disciplines of geology and paleontology, to support his theory. He was also the first to have the crucial insight that the cause of evolutionary change must lie within the reproductive process, which produced random unlimited variations. These random heritable variations placed certain offspring in a favored position to cope with the Earth's constantly changing environment. Darwin postulated that these favored forms were better able to survive and would go on to form species, all members of which would have the new favorable trait. These new species would hold a competitive advantage and would win out over less-favored forms or species in the constant struggle for survival that exists throughout the animal and plant kingdoms. The less-favored forms or species would then diminish in numbers and become extinct. This process was Darwin's

"Natural Selection." Species that were most fit by virtue of a particular trait to cope with an ever-changing environment would displace other less fit or less capable related species. In the universal struggle for existence, the former would survive while the latter would not. To describe this process, Darwin adopted a phrase used in 1852 by Herbert Spencer: "survival of the fittest." However, Darwin's use of the word "fittest" was in relation to a given environment and not on an absolute scale of perfection.[2]

Other aspects of Charles Darwin's life are inherently fascinating. On March 26, 1835, Darwin was heavily bitten by the Benchuca or great black bug of the Pampas.[3] This "kissing bug" carries *Trypanosoma cruzi*, the causative agent of Chagas' disease. Although the disease was not known until long after Darwin's death, it is likely that this infestation produced the lassitude and the heart and gastrointestinal disorders that troubled Charles Darwin throughout his life after the *Beagle*. These symptoms and the resulting semi-invalidism caused Darwin to shun society and other amusements and distractions, thereby giving him the opportunity to concentrate more fully on his work.

Darwin's scientific accomplishments were prodigious and not restricted to *The Origin of Species*. As shown in Table 1, his scientific interests spanned an enormous breadth within botany and zoology. Although some of his secondary works were related to his primary interest in evolutionary theory, others described innovative concepts regarding the formation of volcanic islands and coral reefs, the mechanisms of plant fertilization and reproduction, the power of movement in climbing and insectivorous plants, and landmark studies of the natural history of earthworms and barnacles. In time many of these concepts would become classics.

TABLE I. PUBLICATIONS OF CHARLES DARWIN AND DATE OF FIRST APPEARANCE

JOURNAL OF RESEARCH INTO ZOOLOGY AND NATURAL HISTORY

(DURING THE VOYAGE OF THE BEAGLE)—1839

Sketch of Species Theory—1842

Structure and Distribution
of Coral Reefs—1842

Essay on Species—1844

Geological Observations
on Volcanic Islands—1844

Geological Observations on South
America—1846

Multiple Monographs on Recent and
Fossil Lepadidae and
Balanidae (Barnacles and Acorn
Shells)—1851–1854

Joint Paper with A.R. Wallace on
Evolution and Natural Selection—1858

Origin of Species—1859

Paper on Dimorphism in Primula
(Primroses)—1862

On the Various Contrivances by
Which British and Foreign Orchids are
Fertilized by Insects—1862

Descent of Man—1871

Expression of the Emotions in Man and
Animals—1872

Insectivorous Plants—1875

Climbing Plants—1875

Effects of Cross and Self-Fertilization
in the Vegetable Kingdom—1876

Different Form of Flowers on Plants
of the Same Species—1877

Role of Erasmus Darwin—1879

Power of Movement of Plants—1880

After seriously debating with himself the pros and cons of marriage and its impact on his scientific career, Charles Darwin on January 28, 1939, at age 30, married his cousin, Emma Wedgewood, the daughter of the famous pottery maker Josiah Wedgewood. He rationalized his marriage with the following: "My God, it is intolerable to think of spending one's whole life, like a neuter bee, working, working, and nothing after all. No, no, won't do . . . Marry, Marry, Marry Q.E.D."[2] After marriage, Charles and Emma Darwin, who had 11 children, lived in London for 4 years. They then moved to a country home, Down House in Kent, where he wrote most of his books and articles. Although Darwin's poor health was ascribed to hysteria, anxiety, and hypochondriasis, it is unlikely that a man with the physical stamina, fortitude, and bold spirit he showed during the arduous and adventure-filled voyage of the *Beagle* could be afflicted with these neuroses. The Benchuca and Chagas disease are far more likely explanations for the ill health that formed a backdrop for Darwin's work from the end of 1839 until his death at age 73 on April 19, 1882.

What human qualities best define Charles Darwin? The keynote of his character was simplicity. His wife described him as "the most open, transparent man I ever saw. . . ." Darwin characterized himself as "a great overgrown child" committed to happy endings. He despised cruelty to man and animals, but he recognized that animal experimentation was important for scientific progress, which, in turn, he believed was essential to the betterment of mankind. In the latter part of his life, his religious beliefs centered around natural scientific laws rather than a Creator with unlimited power and compassion. Darwin's self-appraisal of his mental qualities indicated that he "had become skillful in guessing right explanations and devising experimental tests. . . ." He believed he had "no quickness of apprehension or wit. . ." but that he was "superior to the common run of men in noticing things which easily escape attention, and in observing them carefully." He attributed his success in science to "methodical habits, ample leisure from not having to earn my bread . . . and ill health, . . . love of science, unbounded patience, industry in observing and collecting facts, and a fair share of invention [and] . . . common sense."[2] Apart from the ill health, all these qualities would serve an aspiring young vascular surgeon well today.

Despite the turmoil and controversy his theories had created, on his death the greatness of Charles Darwin and the revolutionary importance of his theory to the biologic sciences were recognized. He was likened to Copernicus, Newton, and Faraday and was buried with appropriate honors in Westminster Abbey.

THE CHANGING MEDICAL ENVIRONMENT

Before considering the uncanny relevance of Darwinian principles to Vascular Surgery, it is important to examine some of the forces of change ongoing in its medical environment. All of these threaten the status quo, and some are threatening to the very existence of Vascular Surgery as a specialty. These forces have been fully discussed elsewhere,[4,5] but some bear reemphasis.

The financial support structure for medical care is changing. To restrain escalating health costs, government funding is being curtailed and managed care systems are being introduced widely. These systems provide financial disincentives to use invasive treatments, such as those required by some vascular disease patients. They also tend to place control of the use of these procedures in the hands of generalists rather than the specialists who perform them. All of these changes will make it difficult for the vascular surgeon specialist to function and will increase competition for the reduced dollars that are available to provide care for vascular disease patients.

A second major environmental change is the introduction of technologic improvements that permit less-invasive, more cost-effective treatments. In the vascular disease area this involves a host of endovascular treatments with catheters, balloons, atherectomy devices, stents, stented grafts, and various derivative devices. All of these endovascular treatments involve catheter-guidewire-imaging techniques. All are potentially threatening to vascular surgeons because they may prove equal to or better than open surgical treatments and because they may be administered by nonsurgical interventional specialists with background training in Radiology or Cardiology. Competition of these other specialists with vascular surgeons for patients and limited health care dollars is inevitable. Moreover, interventional radiologists and cardiologists sincerely believe their access to new catheter-based treatments justifies their expanding role in the management of patients who were previously cared for by vascular surgeons.[6–10] Ever-increasing expansion of the workforce in these nonsurgical specialties and decreasing workloads provide further impetus for them to increase their activities in the realm of vascular disease treatment.

A third change in the challenging environment that vascular surgeons face is the re-entrance of general surgeons into the vascular disease treatment field. Decreasing workloads in traditional general surgical procedures, the emphasis on generalist care, and the current antispecialty aura has prompted some leaders in general surgery to advocate broadening the training and role of general surgeons so that they can provide "expertise that at the present time is attributed to various subspecialties, both within and without the realm of traditional general surgery" and can "practice to the fullest extent of the specialty."[11] This is a call to reverse the recent trend for younger general surgeons without special training and certification in Vascular Surgery to *not* perform vascular procedures.[12,13] If this call were heeded, it would negate the purpose of specialized training in Vascular Surgery, namely the provision of better care to vascular disease patients.[14–16] Vascular Surgery came into being as a specialty when it became obvious that general surgeons and cardiothoracic surgeons were not achieving optimal results with vascular operations.[14-16] The improved results of vascular operations, when performed by well-trained surgeons who focus their attention on them and perform them in adequate numbers, has been amply documented by a plethora of studies that are well summarized by Hertzer.[17]

DARWINISM AND VASCULAR SURGERY

To apply the theory and principles of Darwin to Vascular Surgery in its present changing environment demands that we equate a "medical specialty" to a "species." The validity of this equivalence becomes apparent if we recognize that *species* may be defined as a group of individual plants or animals that all have a high degree of similarity, can generally interbreed or reproduce only among themselves, and that show persistent differences from allied species.[1,18] A *medical specialty* may be defined as a group of individual doctors of medicine who, as a result of specialized effort and training in a defined field, have a high degree of similarity in their possession of a special, distinct body of scientific medical knowledge and technical ability that is not possessed in full by other specialists.[19] They concentrate their practice in the well-defined and distinct area of their special knowledge and technical ability, and they have the capacity to reproduce themselves via recognized residency training programs with a defined curriculum and specified case and procedural experiences.[19] Among the objectives of recognized medical specialties and their governing bodies or boards is that they act in the public interest by contributing to the improvement of medical care by establishing qualifications and by evaluating individuals who apply for certification.[20] Establishment of new medical specialty boards "must be based on major new concepts

. . . or substantial advancement in medical science. [They] must represent a distinct and well-defined field of medical practice."[21] Vascular Surgery incorporates a discrete body of knowledge and distinct skills. Many are major new advances. It differs from other specialties, and its members reproduce themselves by recognized residency programs in vascular Surgery. It, therefore, qualifies as a separate *species* or *medical specialty*.

Darwin's theory and principles of evolution and natural selection are particularly relevant to Vascular Surgery if we realize that medical specialties, like species, are engaged in a constant struggle for existence and survival. Our specialty, Vascular Surgery, is in competition with other specialties, Interventional Radiology and Cardiology, for the patients that are the wherewithal to survive and flourish. This competition is rendered more fierce by some of the previously noted forces of change that exist in our environment. These forces will also place us in competition with our more closely related progenitor specialty, General Surgery. The outcome of this competition and struggle for existence will be survival and flourishing with increased numbers for some specialties; for others it will be weakening and diminished numbers; for still others it will mean extinction.

Although the pollyannas may say there will be work for all, medical specialties, like species and individuals, have an irresistible urge to procreate and generally exercise minimal restraint of their excessive reproductive capacity. This leads to unchecked increases in the numbers of individuals within a well-adapted species/specialty, which, as Darwin noted, assures the extinction of less-well-adapted forms that are competing for the same niche in the environment.[1] This niche is defined by food supply and habitat in the case of an animal species and by patients in the case of a medical specialty. Thus the universal struggle for existence inevitably follows from the high rate at which all organic beings and medical specialists tend to increase. Although some suggestions have been made to limit the numbers of medical specialty trainees, these efforts have been limited by antitrust laws and by the obvious incentives, such as prestige and low-cost assistance, that accrue to individuals who direct training programs.

Because a changing environment can and has in the past produced the extinction of innumerable species and some medical specialties and because such extinction is a consequence of poor adaptation to a changing environment, what can Vascular Surgery and vascular surgeons do to assure the survival of their specialty in the present circumstances? They must recognize that their species or specialty is not immutable or fixed by some Creative Power, but must constantly evolve to survive. Moreover, they must realize, as Darwin showed, that transmutation of species is the rule and that several current species or specialties may descend from a common ancestor or progenitor. In the case of surgical specialties, they have all descended from a common progenitor specialty, General Surgery, to become clearly defined and separate specialties. This has been the case for Neurosurgery, Orthopedics, Urology, Plastic Surgery and Cardiothoracic Surgery. It must also be so for Vascular Surgery, if it is to survive. Vascular surgeons must also recognize the applicability of the Darwinian principle that forms that most resemble the common ancestors of several current species or specialties often become extinct as their superior and better-adapted progeny with favorable variations displace them in the endless struggle for existence.[1] Darwin's principle of divergence also applies to medical specialties as well as species. According to this principle, differences between species or specialties that are at first barely perceptible tend to increase steadily, causing the different species or specialties to diverge increasingly in character both from each other and from their common progenitor.[1]

After vascular surgeons recognize that Darwinian theory applies to medical specialties as well as species throughout nature, they must then address three specific issues to minimize the risk of extinction.

VASCULAR SURGEONS MUST ACQUIRE ENDOVASCULAR SKILLS

There are two clear reasons why vascular surgeons must become competent with the catheter-guidewire-imaging techniques that will enable them to perform endovascular treatments. The first is that some of these treatments will prove to be safe and effective and will replace standard open surgical techniques. This is already true for percutaneous balloon angioplasty (PTA) and caval filters. As stents, endovascular grafts, and other newer treatments become perfected, it is possible that 40% to 70% of current operations will be replaced with less-invasive endovascular treatments.[22,23] The survival of Vascular Surgery will depend on the ability of vascular surgeons to adapt and acquire the catheter-guidewire-imaging skills to perform some of the new endovascular procedures that replace vascular operations. If we do not, the need for our services will decrease, we will gradually be replaced, and our numbers will diminish heading toward eventual extinction. As Darwin noted, the "death of a species [specialty] is a consequence of non-adaptation to [changing] circumstances."[1]

It is true that some endovascular procedures are done efficiently by other interventional specialists. Accordingly, it should not be our goal to "take back" diagnostic angiography or the simple catheter-directed treatments that are currently performed mostly by interventional radiologists. To do so is unnecessary and will lead to destructive turf battles.[22,23] However, it is the newer endovascular procedures, many that require surgical as well as endovascular skills, that will replace a large proportion of vascular operations. It is these that vascular surgeons must be able to perform to survive and flourish. Most endovascular grafting and some complex stenting procedures that are performed with an open vascular component are typical examples.

A second reason to acquire endovascular skills is that they can be effectively used to simplify and improve a variety of standard vascular operations. Fluoroscopically assisted thromboembolectomy is an example.[24] Using intraoperative digital C-arm fluoroscopy, a variety of guidewires and double-lumen balloon catheters, it is now possible to perform safer, better thromboembolectomy of even heavily diseased arteries. This technique facilitates over-the-wire passage of the balloon catheter through tortuous, stenotic, clot-filled arteries. It permits visual control of the contrast-filled balloon as it is drawn through diseased arteries to remove the clot, thereby avoiding damage to diseased and normal arteries. It also facilitates complete clot removal and localization and minimally invasive endovascular treatment of significant inflow and outflow lesions.[24]

Intraoperative digital fluoroscopy and catheter-guidewire techniques also facilitate other vascular operations. These techniques enable over-the-wire balloon control of inflow or outflow arteries when infection, scarring, or location renders traditional surgical access difficult. A good example is a case with subclavian artery injury. These techniques allow precise localization of pressure gradients and they facilitate simple endovascular treatment of unexpected lesions. They can also provide more accurate, more complete intraoperative angiograms of arterial reconstructions along with their entire inflow and outflow tracts. With cinefluoroscopy, these improved arteriograms also provide a dynamic index of flow. Vascular surgeons from now on must use these endovascular techniques as an essential survival adaptation in a changing environment. Because the instrumentation is available, we must be able to use it. To do so will render us "fit" to survive. Not to use these techniques is analogous to flying blindly through clouds when good navigational instruments are available. It is a clear path to extinction.

How will current vascular surgeons acquire these endovascular skills? Three steps are involved. One consists of gaining familiarity with endovascular tools, devices, and instrumentation and learning some basic principles regarding their usage, their indications, and their limitations. This information, together with the principles of radiation safety, can be acquired in a Basic Endovascular Techniques Course, which combines didactic teaching with hands-on experience in mock circulatory models. The Society for Vascular Surgery (SVS) and the North American Chapter of the International Society for Cardiovascular Surgery (ISCVS) have made a commitment to conduct such a course to familiarize vascular surgeons with current catheters, guidewires, sheaths, balloons, stents, and intravascular imaging techniques. The first offering of this course preceded this year's Annual SVS/ISCVS Meeting. It was a success and will be repeated if there is a demand for it.

The second step in acquiring endovascular skills is for vascular surgeons to obtain supervised clinical experience. This will be required for the third step, credentialing, which is a local hospital function that will not be discussed further. With regard to clinical experience, some vascular surgeons already have enough to be considered competent. Those that do not can take several pathways to obtain this endovascular patient experience. All involve supervision by a skilled endovascular therapist.

The easiest pathway is for the vascular surgeon to work collaboratively on his or her own patients in his or her own operating room or angiography suite by assisting at or performing the various endovascular manipulations under the tutelage of an experienced colleague, who can be a vascular surgeon, an interventional radiologist, or cardiologist. In such a collaborative setting the interventionalist can serve as a teacher and a consultant if a problem or difficulty is encountered. This training and clinical experience may be provided as part of a healthy and mutually beneficial collaborative relationship, such as an interdisciplinary partnership or a Vascular Disease Center. This is consistent with the observations of Darwin who recognized that one species may be dependent on another. Such species interdependence generally occurs between beings remote in the scale of nature, whereas the struggle for existence will generally be more severe between closely related species.[1] To some extent such specialty interdependence already exists in the current collaborative relationships in which interventional radiologists provide vascular surgeons with high-quality angiograms and vascular surgeons provide surgical resources to interventional specialists for their complications or failures.

When such mutually beneficial relationships are not present within an institution, vascular surgeons must obtain their clinical experience in endovascular techniques at another institution as a trainee for at least 1 to 3 months, depending on the vascular surgeon's level of proficiency and talent, or by performing endovascular procedures with a visiting preceptor who is a skilled endovascular therapist. When either extramural arrangement is required, the SVS/ISCVS should play a major facilitating role by helping to establish a system whereby the necessary experience can be obtained with adequate supervision. The guiding principle in all these arrangements for gaining endovascular experience must be the absolute well-being of the patient. If appropriate skills are not available to one or another member of the team caring for the patient, the procedure should *not* be performed. Whatever pathway is chosen, the degree of endovascular proficiency that the vascular surgeon trainee must attain will depend on the setting in which he will use his new skills. Greater proficiency will be required if the vascular surgeon will not have available immediate interventional consultation and support. Again, the advantages of healthy collaboration between vascular surgeons and other interventional specialists (radiologists, cardiologists, or both) are obvious.

If we accept in the Darwinian sense that current vascular surgeons will have to develop some level of catheter-guidewire-imaging skills to be "fit" enough to survive, it is apparent that we must also assure the endovascular competence of our progeny. To this end, the Association of Program Directors in Vascular Surgery (APDVS) and the Residency Review Committee in Surgery (RRC-S), which oversees training requirements in our specialty, must mandate that Vascular Surgical residency programs provide adequate endovascular training and experience.

MULTIDISCIPLINARY VASCULAR DISEASE CENTERS

The need for vascular surgeons to possess and use endovascular skills has led to the suggestion that vascular therapists of the future be hybrids between vascular surgeons and interventional radiologists. Darwin has pointed out that hybrids between species are generally infertile and weaker than their forbearers and rarely displace them.[1] It is unlikely that the hybrid vascular specialist of the future will be the exception to this rule. There will always be a niche in the medical world for a specialty/species with dominant operative skills to perform complex open operations, despite the need for these individuals to have some degree of endovascular skills. Similarly, there will always be a niche for those with dominant interventional or endovascular skills, despite the advantages of these individuals having some degree of basic open operative skills. The beneficial effects of having both kinds of specialists, each with some degree of these overlapping skills, working together in a true partnership are immediately apparent.[22,23,25] Management of vascular disease patients would be based on what treatment mode was best and most cost-effective rather than on what procedure an individual physician could perform, who saw the patient first, or the resources (operating room or angiography suite) a given physician controlled. Optimal training and patient care would be greatly facilitated and turf issues would be minimized.

The formation of multidisciplinary Vascular Disease Centers in hospitals and medical schools would certainly facilitate true collaborative partnerships between vascular surgeons and other specialists interested in vascular disease diagnosis and management. These other specialists include primarily interventional radiologists but also some interventional cardiologists and those committed to vascular medicine. Some efforts at creating such Centers have already been made in a number of institutions. However, few if any have functioned well.

Because the advantages of such Vascular Centers and other forms of collaborative partnership are so obvious, one wonders why they have functioned poorly and are not already widespread. One reason is the traditional administrative structure in most hospitals and medical schools in which Vascular Surgery is a component of General Surgery and Interventional Radiology is a component of Radiology. Because both of these components are large income producers for their parent departments, there is a natural reluctance to give them the financial or administrative independence to combine and form a new entity linked by their interest in vascular disease rather than their historical derivation from a progenitor specialty. Other reasons are inability to achieve financial integration between specialists, dominance of one or another specialty, and excessive control by the parent Departments of Surgery, Radiology, or Medicine. Underlying all these reasons are the major human motivators, jealousy and greed. Hopefully the enormous benefits of fully integrated Vascular Disease Centers will eventually overcome these negative forces.

To this end, the clear advantages offered by Vascular Disease Centers prompted the Joint Council of the SVS/ISCVS and the Executive Council of the Society for Cardiovascular and Interventional Radiology (SCVIR) to approve a joint statement of support for Vascular Disease Centers. The SVS/ISCVS/SCVIR document recognizes that these Centers, if appropriately structured, will deliver the highest-quality diagnosis, treatment, research, and teaching in vascular diseases. The document mandates that such Centers be comprised of professionals whose primary interest and commitment is to vascular disease patients and that the Centers be administratively independent and co-directed by an interventional radiologist and a vascular surgeon. The document also specifies that all Center patients be cared for on a single integrated service, with management decisions being reached only after joint discussions between members of the two or more involved disciplines. All professional fees accruing to individuals in such a Center would be pooled and distributed on the basis of each individual's overall responsibilities and contributions to the Center. Interdisciplinary training and research would be fostered.

Although resistance to real Vascular Disease Centers based on this document will come from a number of quarters, they will come into being and they will succeed for several reasons. Such Centers will reduce costs. They will provide optimal patient care. They will facilitate the rapid evaluation of new and better treatments. They will minimize the turf battles that might otherwise occur as the result of the shrinking financial support for health care and the introduction of new technologies which cross specialty boundaries. And most importantly, they are intrinsically right because they combine the assets and minimize the liabilities of the many specialties interested in vascular disease management.

RELATIONSHIPS BETWEEN VASCULAR SURGERY, THE AMERICAN BOARD OF SURGERY, AND THE RRC-S

The American Board of Surgery (ABS) and the RRC-S are the governing bodies of General Surgery and Vascular Surgery. The ABS defines the boundaries of General Surgery and administers the examination that certifies general surgeons. The ABS also defines Vascular Surgery and administers the examination for Added Qualifications in that specialty. The RRC-S determines requirements for training and accredits residency programs in both General Surgery and Vascular Surgery. Both the ABS and the RRC-S presently consider Vascular Surgery a component of General Surgery and hold the view that General Surgeons should be trained and qualified to practice Vascular Surgery.

This creates a potential problem or conflict. This stems from the fact that we are training two classes of "vascular surgeons," one which is considered competent by all and holds a certificate to that effect, and a second class that is less well-trained but deemed by some qualified to perform Vascular Surgery—or at least "simple vascular operations." This problem is exacerbated by the fact that the governing bodies for *both* related specialties are the same ABS and RRC-S. This arrangement may be beneficial when the interests of both specialties coincide, e.g., with reimbursement issues or conflicts with other less closely related specialties. However, when the interests of General Surgery and Vascular Surgery diverge, the governing bodies must favor one of two conflicting interests.

One specific example is the recent mandate from the RRC-S that all general surgical residents perform at least 10 aortic cases.[26] Many Vascular Surgery program directors were concerned about this new requirement since aortic surgery is diminishing because of PTA and stenting techniques. This concern was verified by an APDVS survey, which showed that this mandate threatens the viability of at least 28% of Vascular Surgery training programs.[27] The result could be maintenance of the numbers of less well-trained "vascular surgeons," i.e., General Surgeons, at the expense of decreased numbers of well-trained "real" vascular surgeons. How can this be reconciled with the objectives of medical specialization and Specialty Boards "to act in the public interest by contributing to the improvement of medical care . . ." and to ". . . promote and enhance recognition of a single standard in preparation for practice in each specialty"?[20,21] Clearly it cannot on a long-term basis.

The only short-term justification for doing so is the fact that enough well-trained, certified vascular surgeons do not presently exist to perform all the Vascular Surgery procedures required in the United States.[13] It seems reasonable, therefore, to continue to train General Surgeons to fill this gap until adequate numbers of well-trained "real" vascular surgeons can be produced. Consensus was reached on this issue at a recent meeting between leaders of the SVS/ISCVS, the APDVS, and the ABS held on April 29, 1996. At that meeting it was also agreed that the role of the RRC-S, which was not represented, was also important in resolving this problem and related conflicts. It was, however, agreed that better representation of Vascular Surgery, i.e., the APDVS and the SVS/ISCVS leadership, on the RRC-S was urgently required. The meeting ended on a note of optimism that compromise within the present ABS/ RRC-S system could lead to resolution of the conflicting needs of Vascular Surgery and of General Surgery. Hopefully this optimism will be justified by the future actions of our governing bodies.

However, there is little in the history of the relationship between Vascular Surgery and these governing bodies to justify such optimism. Although all vascular surgeons recognize the importance of including a rich Vascular Surgery experience in General Surgery training, issues similar to those present today have received the attention of SVS/ISCVS leaders for more than 26 years.[14–16,28–30] In 1970, when discussing the value of training General Surgery residents in simple vascular procedures, Wylie wondered how many of these programs "would qualify a surgeon for appendectomy who could not remove the right colon . . ."[14] More recently, approval of Vascular Surgery training programs has depended more on the quality of Vascular Surgery training afforded General Surgery trainees than the Vascular trainees themselves.[30] In addition, graduates of adequate independent or freestanding Vascular Surgery training programs have been denied access to the certification process simply because their training was not in an institution with a General Surgery residency.[31] These actions are not consistent with a policy of quickly producing adequate numbers of well-trained Vascular Surgeons, and will tend to maintain the status quo of the two or three class system.

This problem must be resolved soon. The overriding reason is so that *Surgery at large can serve the public better.* Our governing bodies must answer to this call rather than to the parochial interest of any surgeon group or other power base. To reach this goal your leaders in Vascular Surgery can continue our dialogue with the ABS and the RRC-S to obtain better representation for the SVS/ISCVS and the APDVS on these governing bodies. We can maintain steady pressure to see that the needs of Vascular Surgery, our training programs, and, most importantly, the patients we serve are met, so that we can train enough real Vascular Surgeons and provide optimal care to all vascular disease patients—as has already occurred in many other industrialized countries. To maintain a consistent even-handed approach to this problem, the SVS/ISCVS last year formed a Strategic Planning Group that will address this and other issues critical to Vascular Surgery on a long-term basis. Some of these other issues include training in new techniques, workforce analysis, relationships with other specialties and other vascular societies, and vascular research funding.

On all these issues, your leaders can provide analysis and point the way toward resolution. However, problems facing Vascular Surgery may require action and sacrifice and will only be solved if there is consensus and commitment from *all* "real" Vascular Surgeons. In this regard, I define a "real" Vascular Surgeon as a *Specialist in Vascular Surgery or one who has completed at least 1 year of senior level training in Vascular Surgery and vascular disease management, who devotes more than 50% of his or her practice to vascular disease patients, and who performs more than 50 major vascular operations per year.* Although this definition extends beyond the membership of the SVS and ISCVS and it certainly extends beyond the Certificate of Added Qualifications in Vascular Surgery, actions begun in the last year will hopefully lead to ISCVS membership for all such individuals. Clearly the well-being of vascular disease patients will be best served if they are cared for by such specialists.

Charles Darwin has some concluding comments. Vascular Surgery is differentiating from its ancestor, General Surgery. Even though there is a continuing struggle for existence between the two, this will be resolved by the "constant tendency [of] the improved descendants of any one species . . . to supplant . . . the predecessors and original parent" species.[1] Vascular Surgery's descent and separation are inevitable because its members are better adapted, more "fit" by virtue of training and experience to care for vascular disease patients. The divergence of Vascular Surgeons from their ancestral forms will increase with time and be enhanced by increasing special knowledge involving improved operative techniques, vascular biology, noninvasive vascular laboratory techniques, and especially endovascular techniques. Indeed it is likely that endovascular treatments and proficiency in their use will be analogous to the cystoscope in separating Urology from General Surgery, and the pump-oxygenator in separating Cardiothoracic Surgery from General Surgery.

And finally, Darwin would predict that forces of evolution will result in the distinct separation of our specialty, with our own recognized Specialty Board and related Residency Review Committee. That certainly would eliminate much conflict of interest and would probably be best for all concerned, especially for vascular patients.

REFERENCES

1. Charles Darwin, *The Origin of Species* (First published by John Murray, London 1859) New York: Penguin Books, 1968.

2. Sir Gavin De Beer, *Charles Darwin* (Garden City, N.Y.: Doubleday & Co, 1964).

3. Charles Darwin. *Voyage of the Beagle.* (First published as Journal of researchers into the geology and natural history of the various countries visited by *H.M.S. Beagle* under the command of Captain Fitzroy, RN, from 1832 to 1836. Henry Colburn, London, 1839) New York: Penguin Books, 1989.

4. Veith FJ, "The E. Stanley Crawford Critical Issues Forum 1995: the future of vascular surgery in a changing world," *J Vasc Surg* 1996; 23: 894–5.

5. Veith FJ, "The Society for Vascular Surgery: a look at the future," *J Vasc Surg* 1996; 24: 144–7.

6. DeMaria AN, "Peripheral vascular disease and the cardiovascular specialist," *J Am Coll Cardiol* 1988; 12: 869–70.

7. Kinnison ML, White RI, Auster M, et al, "Inpatient admissions for interventional radiology: philosophy of patient management," *Radiology* 1985; 154: 349–51.

8. Katzen BT, van Breda A, "Developing an interventional radiology practice." *Semin Intervent Radiol* 1988; 5: 99–102.

9. Kerlan RK, Marone T, Ring EJ, "The clinical role of the interventional radiologist," *Semin Intervent Radiol* 1988; 5: 103–4.

10. Cook JP, Dzau VJ, "The time has come for vascular medicine," *Ann Intern Med* 1990; 112: 138–9.

11. Ritchie WP Jr., "What the future may hold for general surgery: a position paper of the American Board of Surgery," *J Am Coll Surg* 1995; 180: 481–4.

12. Wheeler HB, "Should vascular surgery become an independent

specialty? implications of data about operative experience," *J Vasc Surg* 1990; 12: 619–28.

13. Stanley JC, Barnes RW, Ernst CB, Hertzer NR, Mannick JA, Moore WS, "Vascular Surgery in the United States: workforce issues—report of the Society for Vascular Surgery and the International Society for Cardiovascular Society, North American Chapter, Committee on Workforce Issues," *J Vasc Surg* 1996; 23: 172–81.

14. Wylie EJ, "Presidential address: vascular surgery—a quest for excellence," *Arch Surg* 1970; 101: 645–8.

15. DeWeese JA, Blaisdell FW, Foster JH, "Optimal resources for vascular surgery," *Arch Surg* 1972; 105: 948–61.

16. DeWeese JA, "Presidential address: vascular surgery—Is it different?" *Surgery* 1978; 84: 733–8.

17. Hertzer NR, "Presidential address: outcome assessment in vascular surgery—results mean everything," *J Vasc Surg* 1995; 21: 6–15.

18. Webster's New World Dictionary. Second College Edition. New York: World Publishing Co, 1970.

19. Annual Report & Reference Handbook—1996. Evanston, II.: American Board of Medical Specialties, Research and Education Foundation, 1996: 106–8.

20. Annual Report & Reference Handbook—1996. p 73.

21. Annual Report & Reference Handbook—1996. p 74.

22. Veith FJ, "Presidential address: transluminally placed endovascular stented grafts and their impact on vascular surgery," *J Vasc Surg* 1994; 20: 855–60.

23. Veith FJ, Marin ML, "Endovascular surgery and its effect on the relationship between vascular surgery and radiology," *J Endovasc Surg* 1995; 2: 1–7.

24. Parsons R, Marin ML, Veith FJ, et al, "Fluoroscopically assisted thromboembolectomy: an improved method for treating acute occlusions of native arteries and bypass grafts," *Ann Vasc Surg* 1996; 10: 201–10.

25. Moore WS, Clagett GP, Hobson RW, Towne JB, Veith FJ, "Vision of optimal vascular surgical training in the next two decades: strategies for adapting to new technologies," *J Vasc Surg* 1996; 23: 926–31.

26. Residency Review Committee for Surgery Newsletter, November 1995.

27. Letter from President (John M. Porter, MD) of the APDVS to RRC-S, April 15, 1996.

28. DeWeese JA, "Presidential address: the vascular societies—how involved should they be?" *J Vasc Surg* 1986; 3: 1–9.

29. DeWeese JA, "Should vascular surgery become an independent specialty?" *J Vasc Surg* 1990; 12: 605–6.

30. Porter JM, "Editorial," *J Vasc Surg* 1993; 18: 100–1.

31. Dardik H, "Training of vascular surgeons: the two-class systems," *J Vasc Surg* 1993; 17: 967–7.

EARLY ENDOVASCULAR GRAFTS AT MONTEFIORE HOSPITAL AND THEIR EFFECT ON VASCULAR SURGERY

Frank J. Veith, MD, Jacob Cynamon, MD, Claudio J. Schonholz, MD, and Juan C. Parodi, MD, New York and Bronx, NY; Cleveland, Ohio; Charleston, SC; and Buenos Aires, Argentina.

Originally printed in the Journal of Vascular Surgery, February 2014.

Edited by Norman M. Rich, MD.

Vascular surgery is very fortunate. It recognized the transition from open surgery to endovascular procedures as treatments for vascular disease early enough to adapt as a specialty. As a result, most vascular surgeons in North America became competent with endovascular techniques, and the survival of the specialty was assured. The endovascular graft program at Montefiore Hospital played a major role in vascular surgery's early recognition of the importance of the endovascular revolution. This article will review the history of this early endovascular graft program and how it influenced the specialty. (*J Vasc Surg* 2014;59:547–50.)

The Montefiore Division of Vascular Surgery had a long-standing interest in aggressive efforts to save lower limbs threatened by gangrene and critical limb ischemia.[1,2] Many of the very distal reconstructive operations were based on unusually fine arteriography performed by our interventional radiology colleagues.[1] In addition, because of the high cardiopulmonary risk of many of our limb salvage patients and the multilevel nature of their arterial occlusive disease, we embraced percutaneous transluminal angioplasty and stenting of iliac and femoral arteries before most other surgical groups.[1,2] In all regards, our Montefiore vascular surgeons were endovascular enthusiasts since the mid-1970s. However, up until 1992, all endovascular procedures except for intraoperative arteriography were performed by the interventional radiologists at our institution with full concurrence and support of the vascular surgeons.

In January 1987, at an International Interventional Meeting organized by Dr Barry Katzen in Miami, one of us (F.V.), who was attending because of interests in percutaneous transluminal angioplasty and stenting, heard a talk on stents and the possible future use of prosthetic graft-stent combinations to treat abdominal aortic aneurysms (AAAs), a concept which had been proposed by Juan Parodi in 1976. This idea and the potential of endovascular treatment of AAAs was a topic of much discussion among the Montefiore vascular group, particularly as a way of treating AAA patients with serious comorbidities. This discussion intensified after Parodi and his colleagues performed the first clinical case on September 7, 1990, and published their initial clinical experience with endovascular aortic aneurysm repair (EVAR) in five patients.[3]

In August 1992, we were asked to care for a 76-year-old man who had a painful 7.5-cm AAA in addition to oxygen-dependent pulmonary insufficiency and severe inoperable coronary artery disease with recurrent ventricular arrhythmias. The patient was mentally alert and wanted his AAA fixed, but was deemed by all who evaluated him to be a prohibitively high risk for an open AAA repair. At that time, EVAR procedures had only been performed in Argentina. Since we had been recently discussing Parodi's work, an endovascular graft repair was quickly considered. The patient appeared to have favorable anatomy for an EVAR procedure, with a long infrarenal neck, a well-defined distal neck, and large straight iliac arteries.[4] So one of us (F.V.) and another Montefiore vascular surgeon, Dr Michael L. Marin, who played a major role in the institution's endovascular graft program, considered journeying to Buenos Aires to learn the procedure and return to Montefiore to perform it.

Dr Parodi was called and indicated that he had no immediate cases planned, but said that he might come to New York City to present his work at our Annual Symposium, and at that time, he might help us perform the EVAR procedure on our patient. Arteriograms and computed tomographic scans were sent to Dr Parodi and then discussed with him by Dr Marin at an interventional cardiology meeting in Milwaukee. At that meeting, it was decided that the patient was a good candidate. However, many logistic issues were left unresolved. One was getting permission from Johnson & Johnson Interventional Systems (JJIS) to use a large Palmaz stent since JJIS had the rights to both Palmaz's and Parodi's patents. The company was concerned that our use of a large Palmaz stent without an Investigational Device Exemption would impair the company's ability to get Food and Drug Administration approval to implant Palmaz-Schatz stents in the coronary arteries.

This issue was extensively discussed at a meeting between Drs Veith and Marin and Marvin Woodall, President of JJIS, and Paul Marshall, Director of New Products for JJIS. The meeting,

FRANK J. VEITH, MD

which was sometimes heated and lasted over 4 hours, took place at a restaurant in the Newark Airport Marriott. After many negative statements from the JJIS team, the issue was finally resolved by having JJIS, which would never let us use their large unapproved Palmaz stent (P 5014), agree to let us use a similar one that was manufactured in Argentina by a company owned by Carlos Sommer.

Next, funds for bringing the Argentinian team to the U.S. had to be obtained. The team consisted of Juan Parodi, Claudio Schonholz, a talented interventional radiologist, and Hector Barone, an engineer who made and assembled the various components of the delivery system and stent graft. Funds for travel and hotel expenses for the team for their stay in New York were obtained from a grant from the James Hilton Manning and Emma Austin Manning Foundation.

Our digital C-arm fluoroscope to be used in the operating room for the procedure was one that had been discarded by an interventional cardiology animal laboratory. When Drs Parodi and Schonholz saw the primitive nature of this instrument, they hesitated to perform the procedure, but were convinced to do so because of their previous commitment and the patient's dire condition.

After obtaining institutional review board approval and with the informed consent of the patient and his wife, his EVAR procedure was performed under local anesthesia on November 22, 1992. A 22-mm knitted Dacron graft was sewn to a large balloon-expandable (Palmaz-like) stent (Fig 1). The endograft, within a large sheath,[3,4] was guided into position fluoroscopically so that the single proximal stent was mostly within the 2.5-cm non-aneurysmal neck of the AAA. The sheath was retracted and the stent deployed by inflation of the balloon on which it was mounted.[4] No distal stent was

266

employed. Despite that, aneurysm exclusion was demonstrated by intraoperative angiography. The prominent AAA pulse was markedly reduced, and the patient's pain was totally relieved. The next morning, the patient had eaten a full breakfast and was sitting up in a chair reading a magazine. He looked far better than any other open AAA repair patient we had ever seen. Postoperative computed tomographic scans and ultrasonography confirmed exclusion of the aneurysm lumen.[4] The patient was discharged 4 days after his procedure, had no abdominal pain, and did well until he died from his cardiac and rhythm problems 9 months later.

This first U.S. EVAR had a profound effect on not only the Montefiore Vascular Surgery Division but also vascular surgery in the U.S. and around the world. The Montefiore vascular surgeons, in collaboration with our interventional radiologists and Argentinian colleagues, embarked on a program of endovascular grafting for the treatment of aneurysms, traumatic arterial lesions, and aorto-iliac and femoral occlusive disease. We used modifications of Parodi's surgeon-made stent grafts or endografts, which consisted of modified commercially available polytetrafluoroethylene grafts with various sized Palmaz stents sewn to them (Fig 2). The stent components of these endografts were mounted on balloon catheters, compressed within a variety of simple hollow tubes or sheaths, then inserted over previously placed guidewires and guided into position under fluoroscopic control. Once in place, the sheaths or insertion tubes were retracted and the stents deployed by balloon inflation. Sometimes, the distal end of these grafts were fixed with a second stent. More often, the distal end of the endograft was fixed within the host artery with an endoluminal hand-sewn suture anastomosis (Fig 3).[5–7]

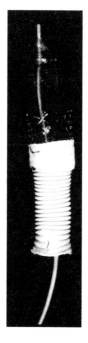

Fig 1. A model similar to the endograft used in the first U.S. endovascular aneurysm repair (EVAR) patient. A Dacron graft was hand-sewn to a large Palmaz-like balloon expandable stent. The compressed stent was mounted on a minimally compliant balloon, which was expanded in the abdominal aortic aneurysm (AAA) neck to fix the proximal end of the endograft to the normal-sized aortic neck.

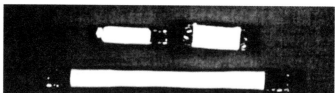

Fig 2. Early surgeon-made stent grafts based on Parodi's concepts.
TOP LEFT, An occlusion device consisting of a Palmaz stent covered by a polytetrafluoroethylene (PTFE) graft closed at one end by ligatures. This was used for occluding the common iliac artery opposite to an aortofemoral or aortoiliac endograft in an abdominal aortic aneurysm (AAA) repair.[5,8] **TOP RIGHT**, A covered stent fabricated by hand-sewing a PTFE graft to a balloon-expandable Palmaz stent, used for treating arterial injuries (eg, of the subclavian artery).[7] **BOTTOM**, A PTFE graft with a Palmaz stent at either end, used for some long iliac or popliteal aneurysms.[10]

We generally used these endografts in patients for whom no other standard endovascular or open surgical treatment option was available because of local or systemic risk factors. These included high-risk AAAs, ruptured AAAs, aneurysms in other locations difficult to reach by open exposures, very difficult limb salvage patients usually after multiple previous failures, and difficult traumatic arterial injuries like subclavian disruptions and arteriovenous fistulas.[5-10] Even in these challenging circumstances, these primitive surgeon-made endografts proved to be surprisingly successful. The procedures proved to be easier and less stressful on the patients undergoing them than we had anticipated, even though our endovascular skills were still not advanced.[5-10]

Because of the relative prominence of our Montefiore vascular group, we were asked to speak on these early endograft experiences quite often. Surprisingly, although we ourselves remained skeptical in our presentations, others hearing them were even more dubious about our results. Indeed, we were often greeted with disbelief, and the opinion of some was that, even if these procedures worked sometimes, vascular surgeons should not be doing them.

Our attitude was just the opposite. We were convinced that vascular treatment was undergoing a revolution: the endo-revolution. We further believed that, if vascular surgeons did not recognize that this was happening and embrace endovascular skills and techniques, they would rapidly be replaced by interventionalists in cardiology and radiology, and vascular surgery would become extinct as a specialty.[11,12]

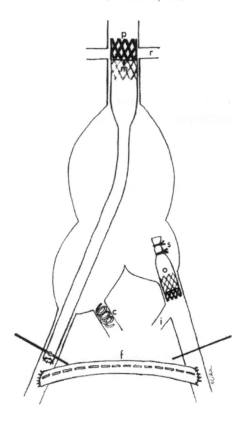

Fig 3. Schematic configuration of a unilateral aortofemoral endograft used for treating complex and ruptured abdominal aortic aneurysms (AAAs). Note the large Palmaz stent (*p*) is partly covered (*m*) and partly uncovered. The open portion of the stent covers the renal arteries (*r*) for secure fixation. An endovascular anastomosis (*e*) fixes the distal end of the endograft within the common femoral artery. The endograft is dilated (not shown) to entirely fill the lumen of the femoral and external iliac artery. When a common iliac aneurysm is present, the ipsilateral hypogastric artery is occluded by coils (*c*). The contralateral common iliac artery is occluded by a covered stent (*o*) closed at one end by ligatures (*s*). The procedure is completed by performing a femorofemoral bypass (*f*).[5,8]

One of us (F.V.) had the good fortune in 1994 and 1996 to be President of two important vascular societies. The theme of the Presidential Addresses before these two societies was that vascular surgeons must recognize the importance of this endovascular revolution and embrace it. Considerable resistance to this was present, at first. Now, however, it is almost universally recognized, and endovascular procedures make up the majority of many vascular surgical practices. Interestingly, even the predictions of an endovascular enthusiast of the late 1990s[12] proved to be short of the mark. With the remarkable creativity of all vascular specialists, it is now likely that more than 90% of the open operations vascular surgeons performed in the mid-1980s will be replaced by endovascular procedures. Even the small proportion of remaining open operations will probably be made simpler or better by using endovascular techniques for a portion of the procedure.[13]

What happened at Montefiore in November 1992 certainly led to an epiphany for our entire vascular group about the nature of vascular treatment in the future. In subsequent years, that epiphany has fortunately spread to the rest of vascular surgery, albeit sometimes slowly. We believe that early recognition and adoption of endovascular treatments by vascular surgeons everywhere will contribute greatly to the survival and prosperity of the specialty.

AUTHOR CONTRIBUTIONS

Conception and design: FV, JC, CS, JP

Writing the article: FV

Critical revision of the article: FV, JC, CS, JP

Final approval of the article: FV, JC, CS, JP

Overall responsibility: FV

REFERENCES

1. Veith FJ, Gupta SK, Samson RH, Scher LA, Fell SC, Weiss P, et al, "Progress in limb salvage by reconstructive arterial surgery combined with new or improved adjunctive procedures," *Ann Surg* 1981; 194: 386–401.

2. Veith FJ, Gupta SK, Wengerter KR, Goldsmith J, Rivers SP, Bakal C, et al, "Changing arteriosclerotic disease patterns and management strategies in lower limb threatening ischemia," *Ann Surg* 1990; 212: 402–14.

3. Parodi JC, Palmaz JC, Barone HD, "Transfemoral intraluminal graft implantation for abdominal aortic aneurysms," *Ann Vasc Surg* 1991; 5: 491–9.

4. Parodi JC, Marin ML, Veith FJ, "Transfemoral endovascular stented graft repair of an abdominal aortic aneurysm," *Arch Surg* 1995; 130: 549–52.

5. Marin ML, Veith FJ, Cynamon J, Sanchez LA, Lyon RT, Levine BA, et al, "Initial experience with transluminally placed endovascular grafts for the treatment of complex vascular lesions," *Ann Surg* 1995; 222: 449–69.

6. Wain RA, Veith FJ, Marin ML, Ohki T, Suggs WD, Cynamon J, et al, "Analysis of endovascular graft treatment for aortoiliac occlusive disease: what is its role based on midterm results," *Ann Surg* 1999; 230: 145–51.

7. Marin ML, Veith FJ, Panetta TF, Cynamon J, Sanchez LA, Schwartz ML, et al, "Transluminally placed endovascular stented graft repair for arterial trauma," *J Vasc Surg* 1994; 20: 466–73.

8. Veith FJ, Ohki T, "Endovascular approaches to ruptured infrarenal aortoiliac aneurysms," *J Cardiovasc Surg* 2002; 43: 369–78.

9. Veith FJ, Lachat M, Mayer D, Malina M, Holst J, Mehta M, et al,

"Collected world and single center experience with endovascular treatment of ruptured and abdominal aortic aneurysms," *Ann Surg* 2009; 250: 815–24.

10. Marin ML, Veith FJ, Panetta TF, Cynamon J, Bakal CW, Suggs WD, et al, "Transfemoral endoluminal stented graft repair of a popliteal artery aneurysm," *J Vasc Surg* 1994; 19: 754–7.

11. Veith FJ, "Presidential address: transluminally placed endovascular stented grafts and their impact on vascular surgery," *J Vasc Surg* 1994; 20: 855–60.

12. Veith FJ, "Presidential Address: Charles Darwin and vascular surgery," *J Vasc Surg* 1997; 25: 8–18.

13. Veith FJ, Sanchez LA, Ohki T, "Technique for obtaining proximal intraluminal control when arteries are inaccessible or unclampable because of disease or calcification," *J Vasc Surg* 1998; 27: 582–6.

JOHN HOMANS LECTURE OF THE SOCIETY FOR VASCULAR SURGERY

A LOOK AT THE FUTURE OF VASCULAR SURGERY

Frank J. Veith, MD, from the Division of Vascular Surgery, New York University-Langone Medical Center, New York; and the Division of Vascular Surgery, Cleveland Clinic, Cleveland. Presented as the Eleventh John Homans Lecture at the Society for Vascular Surgery 2016 Vascular Annual Meeting, National Harbor, Md., June 8–11, 2016.

I would first like to thank Dr. Perler and the Society for Vascular Surgery (SVS) for the singular honor of giving the Eleventh John Homans Lecture. This list of previous Homans lecturers shows why I am humbled by this invitation (Table I). Men like Elkin, Fontaine, Crafoord, Kirklin, Linton, DeBakey, Crawford, Thompson, Hollier, and Moore are the superstars of our specialty. So I am deeply indebted to Bruce Perler for adding me—a maverick from the Bronx—to this list.

First, a word about John Homans—a free spirit and giant in vascular surgery. John Homans was the fifth generation of Boston doctors, dating back to one of his ancestors who was a regimental surgeon in the Continental Army. He was educated and trained at Harvard, the Massachusetts General Hospital, and Hopkins. In 1912 he was picked by Harvey Cushing as one of the first two surgeons at the new Peter Bent Brigham Hospital—where he spent his entire career and became one of the most respected surgeons in the world—largely because of his seminal contributions in venous disease. Dr. Homans was a founding member of the SVS. And he wrote two classic textbooks, one on *Circulatory Diseases of the Extremities* and an even more important *Textbook of Surgery*. This text was the most widely read of its time and was published in six editions and several languages.

John Homans' career was honored by the John Homans Chair of Surgery at Harvard Medical School and the John Homans Lectureship at the SVS. So it is for me the greatest honor to give the Eleventh Homans Lecture, and, at Dr. Perler's suggestion, I have titled it "A Look At the Future of Vascular Surgery."

I realize that predicting the future is risky and that my predictions can be wrong. Also, as Yogi Berra said, "The future ain't what it used to be," and this applies particularly to vascular surgery because the health care system and vascular surgery's position in it has become so different from what it was. However, this topic allows me to tell you what is right and bright about American vascular surgery and the challenges it faces. It also allows me to advise vascular surgery and its future leaders how to help meet these challenges.

Before dealing with the future of vascular surgery, let me touch on the past and the present. In 1992, I had the good fortune to bring Parodi, Schonholz, and Barone to our poor institution in the Bronx, where they, Marin, I, and others performed the first United States (U.S.) endovascular aneurysm repair (EVAR).[1] Seeing the way that case went was an epiphany for me. I had always been enthusiastic about angioplasties, stents, and other endovascular techniques performed by our radiologists. However, that case and our subsequent success with surgeon-made endografts for various arterial lesions made me realize that vascular surgeons had to change or risk becoming extinct.[2]

As a result of that realization, in 1996 I gave my SVS Presidential Address on "Charles Darwin and Vascular Surgery".[2] In that address, I likened specialties to species and indicated that specialties, like species, had to evolve and become different from their ancestors if they were to avoid extinction and survive. I also made three predictions and associated recommendations for future survival adaptations. Two of these recommendations proved to be unworkable or unsuccessful. One proved to be remarkably right.

One errant recommendation was that we work collaboratively with interventional radiologists or cardiologists in dedicated vascular centers.[3] That *Kumbaya* recommendation proved unworkable because of medical tribalism, competitive human nature, and greed. A second recommendation was that vascular surgery become more independent as a specialty, separate from general and cardiac surgery, separate administratively and with an American Board of Medical Specialties (ABMS)-recognized governing board and Residency Review Committee (RRC). A vigorous attempt to accomplish this was made between 1996 and 2007, but was only partly successful.[4] As a result, vascular surgery still remains a subspecialty in North America, although it is not in most other parts of the civilized world.

TABLE I. PREVIOUS HOMANS LECTURERS

Daniel Elkin—1951	Michael DeBakey—1982
Rene Fontaine—1956	Stanley Crawford—1991
Clarence Crafoord—1960	Jesse Thompson—1996
John Kirklin—1971	Larry Hollier—2013
Robert Linton—1976	Wesley Moore—2014

My third recommendation in 1996 fared better. I predicted that 40% to 70% of the open operations we were then doing would be replaced by endovascular procedures.[3] Accordingly, to survive, I recommended that vascular surgeons become endocompetent, learn how to do these procedures, and embrace them. Although this recommendation was greeted with disdain and strongly resisted by many senior vascular surgeons at the time, this resistance was gradually overcome. Our specialty has embraced the endovascular revolution and become endocompetent, and this is why vascular surgery is doing as well as it is today. Indeed, vascular surgeons often lead in developing many evolving endovascular procedures that are currently the standard of care.

As a result, vascular surgery is presently an exciting, vibrant specialty in the U.S. Well-trained vascular surgeons are the only ones who can provide the most appropriate, full spectrum of care for patients with vascular disease, outside the head and the heart, whether that treatment be medical, endovascular, or open. Abundant numbers of patients require our skills. In addition, we use fascinating technology and have good industry relationships. And finally, many patients regard their vascular surgeon as a key doctor who they see regularly. As a result of these advantages, many bright medical students and general surgery residents are choosing to train as vascular surgeons. Vascular surgery should be flourishing.

WHAT HAS BEEN THE EFFECT OF THE ENDOVASCULAR TRANSFORMATION ON VASCULAR SURGERY TO DATE?

Currently, only these vascular conditions or lesions are best treated by open surgery: thoracic outlet and entrapment syndromes, some ascending aorta and arch lesions, a few rare aneurysms not suited for endovascular treatment, some Takayasu lesions, some congenital and genetic aortic and renal artery lesions, some infected arteries and arterial grafts, a rare recurrent or complex lower extremity lesion, some carotid lesions, and some failed endovascular treatments (Table II).

Admittedly there are some vascular lesions for which treatment is still controversial. Carotid stenosis is one such lesion. Presently, endarterectomy, stenting, and best medical treatment all have their advocates in various settings; however, carotid stenting will likely regain increasing favor as technology improves.[5] Another controversial area is the treatment of ruptured abdominal aortic aneurysms (AAAs). Although recent randomized trials show no survival benefits for EVAR, the applicability of these trials is questionable, and EVAR will likely become the standard of care for most ruptured AAAs.[6]

VASCULAR SURGERY IN THE FUTURE

What about the future for vascular surgery in 10 years and beyond?
What changes should we expect?
What are our challenges, and how should we meet them?

First, the easy prediction. *How far will the endovascular revolution go? Will all invasive treatments for vascular lesions become endovascular?* It does not take a soothsayer to realize that more and more vascular lesions will become amenable to endovascular treatment. By 2026, one can predict that 75% to 95% of all vascular lesions requiring treatment will undergo an endovascular procedure (Table III). With the creativity of vascular surgeons and others, this percentage will likely increase. Moreover, all of these treatments will be deliverable via percutaneous approaches.

Does this increasing role for endovascular treatments mean that the day of open surgery is over? Definitely not. There will always be a need for hybrid (open + endovascular) repairs in ~5% of vascular lesions. Cervical approaches to the carotid artery, the need for conduit access, and some open treatments after EVAR are three examples. Also, there will always be a need for fully open surgery in ~5% to 15% of patients requiring invasive treatment, although some of these procedures may be improved by endovascular adjuncts. Open surgical treatment will always be best in some patients with the conditions and lesions I have already mentioned (Table II), although the numbers and proportions of these lesions will decrease as improved endovascular technology and techniques are developed and are proven superior.

How should vascular surgery deal with the decreasing numbers of complex open procedures and who should do them? One solution is to have centers to which these patients are sent and in which vascular surgeons seeking this skill can get adequate open training.

OTHER THOUGHTS ABOUT THE FUTURE

Seminal advances in vascular surgery have always been made possible by advances in other fields, most importantly pharmaceuticals and technology. Heparin, safe contrast agents, and prosthetic vascular grafts are three prominent examples. Similarly, the explosive progress in endovascular treatments was made possible by improvements in digital imaging and the catheter-based technology our industry partners provided.

TABLE II. LESIONS CURRENTLY BEST TREATED BY OPEN SURGERY

Thoracic outlet and entrapments

Some ascending aorta and arch lesions

A few unusual aneurysms

Some Takayasu lesions

Some congenital, genetic aortic, and renal artery lesions

Some infected arteries and grafts

Some recurrent or complex lower extremity lesions

Some carotid lesions

Some failed endovascular treatments

In like fashion, future advances in vascular surgery and vascular disease treatment will depend on advances in other fields. On the horizon are better medical treatments to arrest and even reverse atherosclerosis. Statin drugs are just the beginning and have already decreased rates of heart attacks, strokes, and death.[7] Better use of these drugs will make them more effective, improve our treatments, and help our patients have longer and better lives. Despite this and the possibility of even more effective lipid-lowering with proprotein convertase subtilisin/kexin type 9 (PCSK 9) inhibitors, complications of atherosclerosis will still occur and require our interventions, probably in increasing numbers as our population ages. This ensures a continuing need for the services vascular surgeons provide.

Also brightening the future of vascular surgery and our patients will be advances in the technology that will improve our treatments. This is particularly true with endovascular procedures because of their need for guidance within the vascular system. Glimpses of computer-assisted three-dimensional device navigational tools are already appearing. So also are systems analogous to global positioning within the vascular tree. Radiation will not be required, thereby decreasing hazards to patients and operators. Advances in robotic guidance will also decrease radiation exposure and facilitate device placement. Computer-enhanced simulation will improve training and, when patient specific, will allow procedure planning and rehearsal, thereby improving patient outcomes. Three-dimensional printed models of lesions and blood vessels will contribute to these improvements.

TABLE III. PREDICTED PERCENTAGE OF VASCULAR LESIONS THAT WILL BE TREATED ENDOVASCULARLY BY 2026

LESION	PERCENTAGE
Abdominal aortic aneurysms (AAAs)	90–95
Ruptured AAAs	90–95
Carotid stenosis	75–85
Aortoiliac occlusive disease	90–95
Supra-aortic trunks	90–95
Thoracic and thoracoabdominal aneurysms	85–90
Renal artery stenosis	85–90
Visceral artery occlusive disease	85–90
Infrainguinal arterial occlusive disease	75–90
Traumatic vascular lesons	75–90
Venous occlusive lesions	80–90
Overall	**75–95**

Patient outcomes and the durability of endovascular treatments will also improve with better stent technology. This includes advances in bioresorbable and drug-eluting stents. Similarly, the already promising results of drug-coated balloons will be enhanced. All these devices are complicated with many variable factors. The bottom line is that intimal hyperplasia will be overcome by antiproliferative drugs in all vascular beds once the best way of getting the best drug to the proper location is found. And finally, computer-enabled remote monitoring of flows within grafts and stents will allow corrective treatment before occlusion occurs. Miniaturized piezoelectric sensors are one way to do this.

All these promising new vascular devices and treatments need validation. Their value and cost effectiveness will have to be documented. This will create enormous research opportunities for all academically ambitious vascular surgeons.

So the future for vascular surgery, vascular surgeons, and their patients is bright. There will be exciting new treatments, good research opportunities, and lots of patients needing our attention. However, there are some challenges that vascular surgery must face. How well the specialty deals with these challenges will affect the brightness of its future.

FIRST IS THE CURRENT STATUS OF THE U.S. HEALTH CARE SYSTEM

We live in an imperfect world. We see it in our political leaders who are owned by special interests. We see it in many lawyers who want to translate every untoward effect or bad outcome into a compensatory judgment, with a large share for themselves. We see it in Wall Street and insurance companies that place profit above all else. And yes, we see it in our health care system, in which doctors are able to perform unnecessary procedures for financial gain.

The overuse of outpatient vein centers by those who are not

even vascular specialists is only one example. More importantly, institutional leaders view everything through their prism of diagnosis-related groups (DRGs), relative value units (RVUs), and dollars. Quality care and appropriate care are totally overshadowed by the need to generate money, and poor or unnecessary care is tolerated if providers bring in the patients, the RVUs, and the dollars. There is no easy solution, but clearly, we need an ethical revolution in our country—a return to old-style moral values and behavior. How to do this or how to solve other problems in the U.S. health care system are challenges beyond the scope of this discussion.

A SECOND CHALLENGE IS VASCULAR SURGERY'S ABILITY TO COMPETE WITH OTHER SPECIALTIES

Vascular surgery occupies a competitive niche in the medical environment. Like species in the Darwinian analogy, vascular surgery is competing with other specialties for the institutional resources—or the food and environmental niche—it needs to provide the best care and to survive. These resources include patients, equipment, space, and dollars.

For these essentials, vascular surgery competes, as it always has, with general and cardiac surgeons. General surgeons, however, have become less competitive, but cardiac surgeons have become more in need of work and, thus, more active beyond the heart and thoracic aorta as their open operations are replaced by coronary stents and transcatheter valves. More importantly, as vascular treatments become increasingly endovascular, vascular surgery will be competing with interventional radiology and, importantly, interventional cardiology. The last two specialties have both made contributions to the vascular field and deserve to share in it.

However, the competition with interventional cardiology is and will be intense. Cardiologists do a spectacular job caring for patients with heart disease. However, they also want to expand their role into noncardiac vascular disease, and they have enabling assets. Cardiologists control patients and have a financial incentive to refer to each other. They are capable and much more numerous than vascular surgeons, and they are vigorous in adding to their numbers and aggressively expanding their treatments to areas outside the heart. In fact, many of them have been heard to say publicly that they should replace vascular surgeons. Two exemplary direct quotes from leading cardiologists are: "Vascular surgery is dead, R.I.P.," and "Vascular surgeons, bend over and kiss your butt good-bye."

How can this be? Cardiology is defined in all dictionaries as "the area of medicine that deals with the heart and diseases that affect it" or "the study and treatment of medical conditions of the heart."[8] Nowhere in the definition is the vascular tree mentioned. Nevertheless, in 1988, A.N. DeMaria, then President of the American College of Cardiology, recommended that cardiologists get involved in noncardiac vascular disease treatment because "board certification in the field . . . is nonexistent."[9]

Moreover, interventional cardiologists have the catheter and imaging skills to do so, even though they may lack adequate disease-specific knowledge to go with these skills. This leads them to perform unnecessary carotid and femoral procedures—clearly not good for patient care. Another recent example is their expanding effort to perform endovascular graft repairs for AAAs.

WHAT CAN VASCULAR SURGEONS DO ABOUT THIS?

As individuals or groups, we can practice the best and most appropriate medicine possible and be responsive to patients' needs. These efforts may help us maintain our practice niche. We are, after all, the only specialty devoted solely to vascular disease—its natural history, conservative management, medical treatment, and invasive treatments. Unlike others, we are not just proceduralists.

However, this may have little effect: firstly, because of the diagnosis-related group, RVU, and dollar orientation of institutions, and secondly, because in most institutions we are still considered a subspecialty of general or cardiac surgery, or worse still, a subordinate part of a *heart* and vascular *center*. Administrative control of these centers is rarely in the hands of vascular surgeons. Moreover, when institutional resources, such as angiography suites or hybrid operating rooms are distributed, the interests of vascular surgery are often represented by a general or cardiac surgeon, or worse, a cardiologist.

This limits vascular surgery's ability to get its fair share of institutional resources. The competitive playing field is not level, and vascular surgeons are disadvantaged in the Darwinian struggle to survive. To survive, vascular surgery needs to unify, recognize this inequity, and fix it. This can only be done if all vascular surgeons and the SVS engage vigorously in this issue. We need equal administrative status with cardiac and general surgery in our institutions. Having an ABMS-recognized governing body with its own RRC will help to achieve this improved status. It can also help vascular surgery brand itself as *the* specialty that best takes care of blood vessels and their diseases, something vascular surgery has not done well to date.

Vascular surgery attempted to get such an ABMS-recognized board and associated RRC from 1996 to 2007.[4,10] The main goal of this initiative was to improve patient care and outcomes. The effort had strong support within the SVS but was opposed by the ABMS and some of its member boards. When our application was submitted in 2002, vascular surgery fulfilled the ABMS board requirements. Nevertheless, our application was "denied," and a subsequent appeal was "rejected"—both without explanation. However, vascular surgery did get approval for a "primary certificate" within the American Board of Surgery, and we got improved training with 0 + 5 year vascular surgical residencies for graduating medical students. But vascular surgery still does not have the full recognition of independent specialty status afforded by an ABMS-recognized board and RRC.

Since 2007, vascular surgery has evolved more and is now further differentiated, in a Darwinian sense, from its general surgery ancestor. We have become more endovascular, while general surgery has become more laparoscopic. So vascular surgery is even more qualified now for separate specialty status than it was in 2007.

Because separate specialty status is important to the survival of vascular surgery in our competitive medical environment, the specialty should re-engage in its effort to obtain ABMS approval for such status. Although there may be opposition from several quarters, with strong unity within the specialty, this opposition can be overcome. Other evolving specialties have done it. Vascular surgery can do it too.

Success in this quest will help vascular surgery to flourish and be recognized as the main specialty devoted to patients with noncardiac vascular diseases. Vascular surgery can then fulfill its potential for a brighter future. More importantly, patients and society will be the ultimate beneficiaries.

Thanks for the honor of giving this Eleventh Homans Lecture, and thank you all for your attention.

REFERENCES

1. Parodi JC, Marin ML, Veith FJ, "Transfemoral endovascular stented graft repair of an abdominal aortic aneurysm," *Arch Surg* 1995; 130: 549–52.

2. Veith FJ, "Presidential address: transluminally placed endovascular stented grafts and their impact on vascular surgery," *J Vasc Surg* 1994; 20: 855–60.

3. Veith FJ, "Presidential address: Charles Darwin and vascular surgery," *J Vasc Surg* 1997; 25: 8–18.

4. Veith FJ, "Evolution of vascular surgery and its consequences: the need for an independent American Board of Vascular Surgery," *Vascular* 2004; 12: 149–54.

5. Veith FJ, "Outlook for carotid stenting looks bright," *Interv Cardiol* 2014; 6: 495–7.

6. Veith FJ, Rockman CB, "The recent randomized trials of EVAR versus open repair for ruptured abdominal aortic aneurysms are misleading," *Vascular* 2015; 23: 217–9.

7. Ridker PM, Mora S, Rose L; JUPITER Trial Study Group, "Percent reduction in LDL cholesterol following high-intensity statin therapy: potential implications for guidelines and for the prescription of emerging lipid-lowering agents," *Eur Heart J* 2016; 37: 1373–9.

8. Merriam Webster and Cambridge dictionaries: 2016.

9. DeMaria AN, "President's page; peripheral vascular disease and the cardiovascular specialist." *J Am Coll Cardiol* 1988; 12: 869–70.

10. Stanley JC, Veith FJ, "The American board of vascular surgery: the first 7 years." *Vascular* 2004; 12: 20–7.